SHARING
THE
COVERS

SHARING
THE
COVERS

Every Couple's Guide to Better Sleep

WENDY M. TROXEL, PHD

hachette
BOOKS

NEW YORK

Copyright © 2021 by Wendy Troxel

Cover design by LeeAnn Falciani
Cover photograph © sirtravelalot / Shutterstock
Cover copyright © 2021 by Hachette Book Group, Inc.

Composite Morningness Questionnaire used with permission from the American Psychological Association.

Hachette Book Group supports the right to free expression and the value of copyright. The purpose of copyright is to encourage writers and artists to produce the creative works that enrich our culture.

The scanning, uploading, and distribution of this book without permission is a theft of the author's intellectual property. If you would like permission to use material from the book (other than for review purposes), please contact permissions@hbgusa.com. Thank you for your support of the author's rights.

Hachette Go, an imprint of Hachette Books
Hachette Book Group
1290 Avenue of the Americas
New York, NY 10104
HachetteGo.com
Facebook.com/HachetteGo
Instagram.com/HachetteGo

First Edition: April 2021

Hachette Books is a division of Hachette Book Group, Inc.

The Hachette Go and Hachette Books name and logos are trademarks of Hachette Book Group, Inc.

The publisher is not responsible for websites (or their content) that are not owned by the publisher.

Print book interior design by Linda Mark.

Library of Congress Cataloging-in-Publication Data has been applied for.

ISBNs: 978-0-306-87500-7 (hardcover); 978-0-306-87499-4 (ebook)

Printed in the United States of America

LSC-C

Printing 1, 2021

Contents

Introduction

Love in the Age of Sleeplessness

WHEN I CHOSE MY CAREER AS A SLEEP SCIENTIST AND CLINICIAN, I had no idea how popular it would make me. At parties. On airplanes. At the gym. Everyone wants to talk with a sleep expert. They want advice on what bed they should buy, how to deal with their snoring spouse, what their dreams mean (I have no idea), why they can't get to sleep, why they can't stay asleep, and why they're so tired throughout the day. The list goes on and on. My extremely patient husband, and greatest supporter, takes on his "here we go again" expression when the conversation inevitably veers toward my specialty. But he's a good sport. He knows I love to field these questions. And that's because I truly want to help people sleep better—not just because getting sleep is good for health (it is) but because I believe that if I can help people sleep better, I can help our entire society function better. If we all just slept a little better, we could reduce chronic disease. We could be happier. We could cut down on fatal traffic accidents. We could be more productive. We could get along better. Lord knows, we could get along better.

So I never tire of helping people understand things like how much sleep they need (seven to nine hours for the average twenty-six- to sixty-four-year-old), or what gets in the way of a good night's sleep (our phones aren't helping), or why it's so hard to drag a teenager out of bed in the morning (blame early school start times, not the kid). But the one message about sleep I try to stress more than any other is that your ability to get a good night's sleep affects the quality of your most precious relationships, and the quality of those relationships affects your ability to sleep. Because of that, working to improve your relationships can improve your sleep, and working to improve your sleep can improve your relationships.

You see, I'm a bit of an oddity in the professional world of sleep. First, I am both a sleep researcher and a sleep therapist. Those combined facts don't by themselves make me particularly unusual. There are many others like me in those respects. While I love the academic/research side of my profession and can completely nerd out with it, maintaining a clinical practice helps keep me grounded and gives my research purpose. What makes me odd compared to my peers is that in my research and in my clinical work, I look at sleep through an interpersonal lens. That is, I view sleep as inherently a social behavior. Why is that odd? Because over the past sixty years, most of the groundbreaking research in sleep science has come from studies of people sleeping alone in a laboratory, under tightly controlled conditions, free from disruptions, and as isolated as possible. Consequently, the majority of therapeutic sleep interventions treat sleep issues as an individual's problem. While there is a lot to learn about how individuals sleep, and there is a lot that individuals can do (and likely need to do) to improve their sleep if they are suffering, our historical approach to both the research of sleep and the treatment of sleep disorders has failed to recognize that, for the majority of us, sleep is a shared experience.

Sleep doesn't occur in a lab. It occurs in our bedrooms. A lot of other things also occur in our bedrooms. Some things we like — the sex, the cuddling, the pillow talk, the bonding. Some things we don't like — the lack of sex, the late night arguments, the sheet-stealing, and children (whether human or the furry kind) wedging themselves between us. If we're going to help people improve their sleep, we need to treat it in terms of the real-world contexts in which it happens (or doesn't happen).

In its annual survey of the nation's sleep habits, the National Sleep Foundation found that 61 percent of adults sleep with a bed partner and one-quarter to one-third of adults reported that their intimate relationship has suffered as a result of their own or their partner's sleep problems. You probably don't need a national survey to tell you this (as virtually everyone who has ever shared a bed with another human being for any consistent period of time can tell you): when sleep is shared, your sleep problems are your partner's sleep problems, and vice versa. Scientific neglect of the coupled nature of sleep has led to a number of misconceptions and paralyzing stigmas about the meaning of the marital (or otherwise shared) bed, which I'll uncover throughout this book. It's also led to a nation of sleep-deprived couples.

I've witnessed the interconnected nature between sleep and relationships directly in my clinical practice as well. The vast majority of my practice has been focused on the treatment of insomnia, because unfortunately there is no shortage of people struggling with insomnia. It's the most common sleep disorder, and it can be quite brutal. There is, however, a severe shortage in trained providers in the most evidence-based treatment for insomnia, known as cognitive-behavioral therapy for insomnia—the type of treatment I provide.

Sometimes insomnia is the result of stress at work. Sometimes it's the strain of parenthood. Sometimes insomnia rears its ugly head when a relationship is on the rocks or ending. The potential causes of insomnia are plenty and almost always a combination of factors. The most effective treatments, though, involve changing thoughts and behaviors about sleep, and in many cases, the bed partner is along for the ride, like it or not.

The classic clinical scenario that I see repeatedly goes something like this. My patient—often, but certainly not always female, as women are about twice as likely to have insomnia than men—struggles nightly to fall asleep and stay asleep, while, with growing resentment and downright animosity, she watches her partner blissfully and effortlessly sleep through the night. While she structures her world around when and if she might be able to sleep better and constantly thinks about the consequences of not sleeping well (incidentally, this is in fact part of the problem that we address in treatment), her contempt grows as she watches her partner achieve her elusive goal without even trying. The nerve.

While most people initially come to me individually to treat their condition, it has often morphed into somewhat of a couple's therapy experience, as I work with the couple to find strategies to negotiate and compromise to enhance their shared sleep. It's important to acknowledge that there are definitely things that each of us can do as individuals to improve our sleep, but if we ignore the role of our relationship in our sleep (or vice versa), we may be missing a critical part of the treatment equation.

RELATIONSHIPS MATTER

For many of us, developing and maintaining healthy relationships is a perennial priority. In fact, eight out of ten adults say having a successful marriage is one of their top goals in life, if not the top. We spend a lot of time, money, and energy thinking, talking, and reading about how we can achieve relationship harmony. It's no wonder that the relationship self-help industry is a booming multibillion-dollar business. Just walk through any self-help section of your favorite bookstore, and you will find shelves filled with books on how to improve your relationship. But while we've been pining away for solutions to optimize our relationship health, we've systematically neglected to consider a crucial one-third of our lives that has a direct impact on the quality of those relationships: sleep. In traditional marital vows, we speak the words "for richer, for poorer" and "in sickness and in health"—dichotomies that represent the promise of a lasting relationship through the many cycles of life. But what about the most immediate cycle—day and night—the twenty-four-hour rhythm that our bodies run on, punctuated by roughly sixteen hours of wakefulness and, if we are lucky, eight hours of sleep?

SLEEP MATTERS

Over the past ten years, you may have noticed a similar proliferation of books on how to achieve the increasingly elusive night of good sleep. These traditional relationship and sleep self-help books have, by and large, completely ignored each other's existence. When it comes to the bedroom, relationship researchers often talk about sex but rarely if ever about sleep. Yet sleep occupies about one-third of our lives. Proportionally, that's a major part of our coupled existence—much more so than sex. Think about your own relationship. What other time do you regularly spend seven to nine hours (ideally) in close physical proximity to your partner? The shared sleep experience is arguably the most concentrated period of time in which couples are actually together in a shared physical space. It's even been said that sleep is the new sex. Everyone's talking about it, wishing they had more of it, and feeling envious of friends and coworkers who seem to get plenty of it all the time. But if sleep is the new sex, then why do we know so little about what it actually means to "sleep together" (in the literal sense, not the biblical one)? Sleep experts have largely neglected to consider the impact of the bed partner, just as relationship experts have largely neglected to consider the third of couples' lives spent asleep. It's the coupled nature of sleep that drove me to write this book, with the goal of helping you improve your sleep and your relationships at the same time.

Before we get into how sleeplessness manifests itself in couples, let's review how individuals are faring on the sleep front, starting with the fact that about one in three American adults regularly gets less than the seven to nine hours of sleep that doctors and sleep scientists recommend. Our culture is steeped in this entrenched belief that more work is always better and that sacrificing sleep is a necessary, even noble feat in the pursuit of personal betterment and success. The saying "sleep when you're dead" is so integral to today's culture that it has inspired songs by bands from Bon Jovi and the Cure and by singers from rocker Warren Zevon to country artist Jason Michael Carroll. This mortally misinformed belief has wreaked havoc on many a mind and body. Rather than marching us toward personal growth and success, it may be marching us more quickly to our graves.

Sleep loss and sleep disruption are directly linked with increased risk for mental health problems, such as depression and suicide; physical health problems, including our expanding waistlines, heart disease, and diabetes; Alzheimer's disease; and even early death (so I guess, here's your opportunity to sleep).

As a society, we typically think of sleep loss and sleepiness as personal problems, but the consequences of poor sleep go well beyond the individual, affecting our closest relationships, our productivity, and even our economy. My brilliant economist colleague, Marco Hafner, along with our RAND colleagues and I showed that sleep loss costs the US economy $411 billion per year, which is 2.28 percent of the GDP. These economic losses were largely driven by the 1.2 million working days that are lost as a result of an unproductive or absent, sleep-deprived workforce as well as the increased mortality rates associated with sleep loss. We observed similar economic losses in other sleep-deprived countries, including Japan, Germany, the UK, and Canada.

Our economics report made a big splash in the news, with headlines in every top-tier media outlet around the globe. Of course, it's wonderful to see our work having such a significant impact, but I find it ironic that it took us attaching a dollar amount to sleep loss for the world to start waking up to the consequences—as if the health consequences were not enough. Far from the need for sleep being just a personal problem or a sign of weakness, these data confirmed that the consequences of sleep loss are a societal problem.

The funny thing is, this tremendously successful and ongoing collaboration between a sleep scientist (me) and an economist (Marco) was born out of Marco's personal battle with sleep, which took a huge hit on his marriage and the rest of his life.

Like most economists, Marco's work was focused on trying to understand the economic impact of things people do during the two-thirds of our lives when we are awake—we go to work, we provide labor, we consume, we save (well, some of us), and we invest.

But then Marco's daughter was born. "She was the worst sleeper ever," he recalls. "For the first year or more of her life, she woke up every hour throughout the night."

Marco had never really thought that much about sleep or sleep loss because it had never been a big deal. As a university student, when schoolwork forced him to stay up all night, he just caught up on his sleep once the deadline had passed. But with his daughter, he became the poster child for sleep deprivation.

"It literally changed my personality," he says. "I consider myself a pretty sociable person, and I genuinely like being around people. But I became this completely antisocial person."

In addition to directing his wife to turn down social events, he shut down on the communication front, which had previously been a strength. Not only did small talk seem like too great an effort, he lacked the motivation to even talk to his wife. When he did summon the energy to speak with people, a sarcastic, demeaning tone colored the exchanges. "Unfortunately, my wife bore the brunt of that," he says.

This normally witty guy completely lost his sense of humor as well as his perspective: "Suddenly, I only saw the negative side of things. My patience was down to nothing, and I realized for the first time that I have quite a temper—getting mad at my wife or kids for the silliest things that weren't even their fault."

The challenges he experienced because of sleeplessness spilled over into the rest of his life. He'd drive to work on little sleep, arriving at the office in a fog, with little understanding of how he made it to the office. At work, he struggled to get tasks done. Worse yet, his mental clarity and focus, which had been his bread and butter, allowing him to think through and solve problems in creative and innovative ways, were reduced to mush. Not surprisingly, as his productivity tanked, the job front got more stressful as well, which only accentuated the anxiety and depression he was feeling.

He started to think, "If my professional and personal lives are suffering this much because of lack of sleep, then what does this mean in the big picture?"

Billions of people worldwide, like Marco, are not sleeping enough. Add up the consequences of sleep loss for those people, and you get a whopping hit to the global economy, which is exactly what our report found. Of course, as I mentioned earlier, most people don't sleep alone. So more often than not, they share their sleep problems. That not only multiplies the economic costs, it takes a toll on their relationships as well, just as it did for Marco and his family. But it's also true that relatively small changes can make a big difference. For example, our analysis showed that if those who sleep under six hours a night increase their sleep to between six and seven hours a night, this could add $226.4 billion to the US economy. Marco also learned, as you will learn in this book, that there is a lot individuals and couples can do to improve their sleep, and doing so can have profound results for personal and interpersonal happiness.

I have spent my career seeking to understand how sleep and relationships are related, and how they collectively and interactively influence how we feel, how we behave, our health, and our survival. What my research and that of others has shown is that sleep and relationships are bidirectionally linked. In other words, problems in either the sleep or the relationship domain can lead to a vicious and mutually reinforcing cycle. On the other hand, we have an opportunity to flip that cycle and turn it into a virtuous one. Perhaps by focusing on how our sleep problems affect not just ourselves but also the quality of our relationships, we can shift some of these cultural attitudes that see sleep loss as a badge of honor, and instead we can view sleep as a vital pillar of our personal health and well-being, our productivity, and our relationships.

When I set out to write this book, the world was a very different place from what it is today. I was over halfway through writing the book before the SARS-CoV-2 (i.e., COVID-19) came along to upend everything. When the initial emergency declarations hit and we all went into lockdown, my initial thought was, "Well, now at least, I will really have some time to buckle down and focus on finishing this book." Like many who had initial lofty aspirations of using the lockdown to become super-productive, super-fit, a super-baker, or super-whatever, I quickly realized that despite the fact that my calendar was suddenly completely barren, the stress, turmoil, and uncertainty of the times got in the way of my fantasies of manic productivity. Ultimately, what got me out of my wallowing and back to the grind of writing was the stories I heard from friends, from clients, and in media reports that shined the spotlight on the vital role of healthy sleep and healthy relationships, and how the pandemic has challenged them both. During Zoom calls with colleagues, when an errant spouse or child wandered into the background, or when friends with small children talked about the stress of balancing their and their partner's workload while all of a sudden also trying to homeschool their kids, or when I heard the countless stories of the sleepless nights and wacky coronavirus-related dreams that seemingly everyone was having, I realized that perhaps now more than ever sleep and relationships were ready for their moment.

Introduction

Our well-being, individually and as couples, has taken a shock to the system like most of us have never seen before. The stress of it all, and the losses and disappointments we have experienced, while clearly different for everyone, has put pressures on our relationships and on our sleep. They say that when China came out of lockdown, the divorce rate skyrocketed; reports of domestic violence are on the rise in the US and worldwide. I don't know what's going to happen in the United States with divorce rates, or marriage rates, for that matter, but I do believe that this pandemic has exposed how fundamental our relationships and our sleep are to our health and well-being. They are truly the cornerstones of health, and yet we so often take them both for granted. If COVID-19 has made either more difficult for you, or if COVID-19 has made you realize the vital importance of healthy sleep and healthy relationships, I hope you find in these pages something that helps. I'd like to think you will.

Be safe. Sleep well. Love heartily,
Wendy

How to Read This Book

IF YOU'RE IN A RELATIONSHIP, AND IF YOU OR YOUR PARTNER OR BOTH of you are struggling with your sleep, this book can help. If you and your partner are struggling in your relationship, this book can help, too. This book will give you tools to work on your sleep individually and collaboratively. It will also give you tools to work on your relationship. This book will not solve all of your relationship or sleep woes, particularly if they are severe, and it should not be considered a replacement for seeking professional help if the situation calls for it.

Each chapter in this book explores a different aspect of the shared sleep experience. I'll expose you to a number of studies to help you better appreciate the science of sleep and the coupled nature of it. I'll also share a number of stories along the way—stories from my clinical practice and elsewhere that help provide some important real-world context for the academic research. Every chapter ends with a contribution to your Shared Sleep Action Plan—a simple exercise you and your partner can do together to work on either your sleep or your relationship or both. (Remember, working on either is working on both.) My hope is that, when you're done with this book, you and your partner will have had the important conversations about what you both want for that third of your life together that you will spend sleeping.

This book is meant for "every" couple. However, when it comes to reporting the existing evidence base, I am limited by the science that exists. Sadly, this is lacking diversity in several areas, including inclusion of same sex or mixed gender couples. The good news is that the basic challenges that couples face in their shared sleep experience and the strategies to overcome them, are universal. Nevertheless, we do need more research (and funding to support it) that represents "every" couples' sleep experience.

It's also important to acknowledge that circumstances differ, so certain suggestions I offer may not be available to some couples (e.g., having an extra bedroom or having access to good clinical care). Unfortunately, sleep problems are more prevalent in groups that are more socially and economically disadvantaged. It is easy to appreciate how a cramped living space, a noisy or unsafe neighborhood, and working multiple jobs, including shift work, could create added challenges for a good night of sleep (although I recognize that for shift workers and others, "a good night of sleep" means something a bit different). This is a truism that we need to face as a society and strive to change with policy and action, so that healthy sleep is not a luxury reserved for those who can afford it. While, sadly, there is no easy fix for some of the challenges, even small changes can make a big difference to our sleep. Most of the strategies covered in this book are more about how you and your partner communicate and relate with one another and less about things you need to have. I truly believe that effort to work on your sleep and your relationship can benefit both, and many of the tools for doing so are readily available for any couple in any context, should you choose to use them.

When I wrote this book, I imagined partners lying in bed together at the end of the day reading the book and completing the Shared Sleep Action Plan together. I'm going to keep imagining that. You, of course, can read this book however you want. And while I wrote it assuming you'd read all the chapters in order, I recognize that you may have specific interests and goals for you or your partner's sleep. If you'd rather hop around, you may use the following chapter outline to explore a high-level description of each chapter so you can determine which ones interest you most.

CHAPTER 1: SLEEPING TOGETHER (OR NOT)

What does it say about your relationship if you and your partner sleep in separate beds? That depends. This chapter explores what we actually know about the costs and benefits of sleeping together or apart and why most people prefer to sleep with their partner even though, by objective measures, people tend to sleep worse when sharing a bed.

CHAPTER 2: SLEEP AS IF YOUR RELATIONSHIP DEPENDS ON IT

Is sleep really that important to your relationship? Yes. This chapter shows just how the quality of your sleep and the quality of your relationship are deeply interconnected.

CHAPTER 3: A TOXIC DANCE

When we're sleep-deprived, we're bad partners. When we're bad part-ners, we're sleep-deprived. It's a toxic dance. This chapter shows just how sleepless nights can lead to relationship strife.

CHAPTER 4: A VIRTUOUS CYCLE

For every behavior that can derail a relationship, there's an alternative behavior that can bolster it. Practicing these behaviors can improve your sleep. Getting good sleep can make it easier to practice these behaviors.

CHAPTER 5: HIS, HERS, AND OUR SLEEP

From biology to behavior, men and women experience sleep differ-ently. Understanding these differences can help you and your part-ner better accommodate each other's unique needs when it comes to sleep. This chapter discusses how and why men and women sleep differently, how these biologically and socioculturally based dif-ferences in sleep can create co-sleeping challenges for heterosexual couples.

CHAPTER 6: ROOM FOR MORE?

Do babies make it hard to sleep? Duh! This chapter gives you prac-tical guidance for navigating the inevitable sleep pain that comes when you bring kids into your family.

CHAPTER 7: ARE WE IN SYNC?

Does it matter that your partner wants to go to sleep at nine and you want to burn the midnight oil? It could. This chapter explores circadian rhythms, a primary intrinsic driver of differing sleep-wake patterns, and a key driver of relationship challenges when mismatched pairs share a nest.

CHAPTER 8: IN SICKNESS AND IN HEALTH

This chapter integrates research focused on the impact of mental and physical illness on sleep, including sleep in the context of caregiving, as caregivers are among the highest-risk groups for sleep deprivation.

CHAPTER 9: SNORING AND OTHER SHARED SLEEP STRUGGLES

Insomnia, obstructive sleep apnea, restless legs syndrome—there are so many ways sleep can go wrong. This chapter focuses on the most prevalent clinical sleep disorders and will provide perspectives on how the disorder can affect both partners' sleep and the quality of their relationship.

CHAPTER 10: NEGOTIATING THE NIGHT

You both need to sleep—for yourselves and for your relationship. This final chapter helps couples identify their individual and collective needs and provides a series of concrete best practices to help you improve your sleep, your health, and the quality of your relationship.

chapter one

SLEEPING TOGETHER (OR NOT)

J ENNIFER IS A TWENTY-EIGHT-YEAR-OLD WRITER FOR AN ONLINE media outlet. I met Jennifer because she was writing an article about why it might not be such a bad thing for some couples to sleep in separate beds. Before long, Jennifer revealed to me that this interview wasn't just research for her article. It was personal. She and her partner, Steve, had made the decision to sleep apart. While they made the decision jointly (while in bed no less), Jennifer couldn't help wondering if their choice suggested their relationship was in trouble. For them, it was an issue of timing. She, as a writer and as a natural night owl, often got her biggest burst of creativity and productivity after ten p.m. Steve, on the other hand, who worked a more traditional day job as an engineer, was ready to conk out around ten p.m. and would get increasingly frustrated with Jennifer's late-night pitter-patter on her keyboard as they lay together in bed. She, in turn, felt resentful because she felt he was stymieing her most creative time of the day. Both were resistant to even having the conversation about sleeping apart. It felt so old school, like a scene from *I Love Lucy*—hardly the image they had of themselves as passionate and in-love twentysomethings.

At first, Jennifer explained to me, they dabbled in sleeping apart. On occasion, particularly when Jennifer had a major deadline and needed to stay up late to write, she would preemptively decide to sleep in the guest bedroom. Initially, neither Jennifer nor Steve was willing to admit that this sleeping strategy actually worked better for both of them. But after dabbling as solo sleepers, they started to realize that when Jennifer slept in the other bedroom, they were both happier and less resentful, and they could enjoy their time together in bed, particularly on the weekends, when there wasn't the pressure of their incompatible sleep schedules. So what started as dabbling has become their norm. And it works for them. Jennifer and Steve made the right decision for themselves and for their relationship. I could feel Jennifer's relief through the phone when "the sleep expert" told her so. She had her story and her validation.

Friends of mine, Evelyn and Jack, a couple at the other end of the age spectrum, both in their seventies and married for over thirty years, couldn't imagine such an arrangement. I recently visited them in their *Architectural Digest*–worthy house, with its vaulted ceilings and panoramic views, and every inch of the roughly five thousand square feet of living space impeccably decorated. Then we arrived at the bedroom, and I had to laugh. In the center of their oversized and stunningly beautiful bedroom in their high-end custom home, was the puniest bed I've ever seen. In disbelief, I had to ask, "Is that a double bed?" Indeed it was. This was the mattress-related equivalent of "Where's the beef?" Not only have they always shared a double bed throughout their thirty-plus-year relationship, but Evelyn sheepishly admitted that they almost always fall asleep holding hands or having an arm draped across the other, with clothing optional. She went on to explain that, "Throughout our careers, Jack and I have had to travel a lot. We both had previous marriages too, and learned that so much travel can take a toll on your relationship over time. I think that's why, for Jack and I, when we are home together, we've really made it a priority to maximize the time we spend together so we can stay connected. And nighttime is a big part of that." For both of them, physical contact has been key to their sleep and relationship success.

Over the years, there's been one question that's kept cropping up again and again. It's this: "Is it bad if my partner and I sleep apart?" Couples of all types, heterosexual, same-sex, young, old, long-time bed partners, and newlyweds alike—they've all asked me this very question.

Underneath the question is the desire for some sort of validation, from me, the "expert," that their choice to sleep apart is okay and not the death knell of their relationship. I've always been struck by this need to seek external validation for what is arguably one of the most intimate behaviors a couple can share. But at the same time, I completely understand. We're taught to believe that a couple who sleeps together stays together. We make assumptions that couples who sleep apart must be on hard times—perhaps even assuming (rightly or wrongly) that their relationship is a loveless, sexless mess. We've even created a super judge-y name for when couples choose to sleep apart: sleep divorce. If that couple is you and your partner, it can make you question the very viability of your relationship. Are you being judged? Are those judges right?

The two couples whose stories I used to start this chapter illustrate an important point. Every couple has to find what works for them and for their relationship. The truth is that Jennifer and Steve couldn't possibly make it work sleeping in the buff while spooning on a double bed. Evelyn and Jack couldn't imagine saving their night-long canoodling for the weekends while heading to separate rooms during the week. Each might think the other couple's decision is weird, but that doesn't really matter. What matters is finding what helps you and your partner both get the sleep you absolutely need while maintaining intimacy, partnership, and health. Of course, doing so is easier said than done.

THE STIGMA OF SLEEPING APART

There is a huge amount of pressure around the meaning of the marital or otherwise shared bed, but this is largely a socially constructed belief system, not science-based. Sleeping apart is not necessarily a sign of a failing relationship. Of course, sleeping together does not guarantee a successful one. (If only it were that easy!) And that term "sleep divorce"? I hate it. The idea that "sleep divorce" is some sort of benign, cutesy phrase to capture a growing societal trend just feels wrong to me. Under no circumstance is the term "divorce," applied in the context of a relationship, a benign term—it's fraught with meaning, connoting relationship rupture and turmoil. What we are really talking about is a couple's decision to make the choice that's right for them when it comes to a critically important health behavior. For that reason, I won't use that phrase going forward. I hope you won't either. Think of it as forging a *sleep alliance* with your partner, not a sleep divorce, or in the words of journalist Jessica Goldstein, "unconscious uncoupling."

There are reasons to spend the night together, including emotional connection, security and comfort, health concerns, or the sense of getting better rest. There are also reasons not to, like different sleep-wake schedules or preferences for sleeping environments (your partner is always hot; you're always cold), children (including the furry kind), sleep disorders, or maybe one of you is just a really light sleeper, who wakes up the minute the other person rolls over. Suffice it to say, if you're not sleeping well together, different arrangements might work better.

Remember: sleep makes up about one-third of your entire life; proportionally, that's a major part of your coupled existence. How you and your partner decide to spend that one-third of your lives is something you have to decide for yourselves. As with most major decisions in a relationship, the healthy strategy comes through shared decision making and open and honest communication. But the point is that it's not sleeping arrangements that decide whether a couple can have a strong, passionate, and love-filled relationship. It's the couple who decides that.

It's a shame that, rather than having open and honest communication about what's working and what's not working in the bedroom (and this goes well beyond the time spent engaged in sex), many couples are operating on a sense of "shoulds," based on socially prescribed norms, which are subject to change. And the truth is that the expectation that happy couples sleep together is a rather modern perspective. Throughout Western history, the pendulum has shifted back and forth from stigma attached to sleeping together versus sleeping apart. Understanding the historical, social, and cultural patterns in couples' co-sleeping behaviors provides the necessary context to start breaking down the tired myths about sleeping together (or not) that pervade our culture and that can leave many couples feeling at best uncertain, and at worst ashamed, about their sleeping arrangements.

CUDDLING UP ACROSS THE AGES:
A VERY BRIEF HISTORY OF SLEEPING TOGETHER (OR NOT)

From an evolutionary perspective, one could argue that sleep is a really bad idea. Think about it. You're lying down, semiconscious, and with eyes closed. In other words, easy prey for a hungry predator. Think of all the time that is wasted while sleeping, putting us in this highly vulnerable position. And yet we literally cannot survive without sleep. As one of the legends in sleep, Allan Rechtschaffen, has said, "If sleep doesn't serve an absolutely vital function, it is the biggest mistake evolution ever made." I couldn't agree more.

Our social nature likely evolved in parallel or in support of the vital function of sleep. After all, we derive safety in large part from our connections with others. Historian A. Roger Ekirch wrote that night was "man's first necessary evil," inspiring widespread fear, particularly in pre-industrial (i.e., before artificial light) societies. According to Ekirch, "Never did families feel more vulnerable than when they retired at night. Bedmates afforded a strong sense of security, given the prevalence of perils, real and imagined—from thieves and arsonists to ghosts, witches, and the prince of darkness himself." This fear of night is likely hardwired into our DNA—and so is one of our primary coping responses to fear: connection to others. Both the fear and the response have persisted in postindustrial societies as well, though the risks of being eaten or attacked in our sleep are vastly lower than for our ancestors. Nevertheless, at least in contemporary Western cultures, we have generally settled on sleeping with a single bed partner. This partner is typically a romantic mate rather than a child or other bedmate. But this hasn't always been the case.

Since the Middle Ages (spanning about the fifth to fifteenth centuries) in European society, beds were communal. Bed sharing, not just with romantic partners but also with children, other relatives, animals, and even total strangers (e.g., for travelers staying at an inn), was considered both normal and practical and provided some basic survival necessities, like security and warmth, not to mention that, particularly for more modest homes, a shared bed was less costly than having multiple beds and took up less space, which was at a premium. In addition to serving these practical purposes, communal sleeping arrangements also provided psychological benefits, in part because many of the social rules and norms that governed the day time vanished or at least faded when the lights went down. To be sure, there were still rules in bed, particularly when it came to who got to sleep where. An Italian proverb advised sleepers, "In a narrow bed, get thee in the middle," as the middle was the place of greatest warmth, whereas the edges of the bed were reserved for visitors or strangers—as far from the women as possible. But even with such rules, the shared bed offered a leveling of the playing field across the usual social hierarchy. For example, a "master" or "mistress" might share a bed with a servant or maidservant, respectively, and in a patriarchal society wives were somewhat more empowered to speak their minds to their husbands relative to daytime. In the 1768 diary entries of John Eliot of Connecticut, he bemoans his wife's nighttime rants, in which she keeps them both awake "raking up the old stories about the first and second wife, first and second children, etc." (Perhaps we aren't so different from our ancestors after all.)

But pillow talk of the past was often far from contentious. The talk that occurred in bed ranged from deeply personal and revealing to boisterous and funny—including the telling of bawdy jokes among bedfellows. What struck me most about reading these historical texts and speaking with historian Roger Ekirch is how different our prebedtime rituals are today, even when bedsharing is reserved for romantic partners. How much have we lost in terms of our opportunity to strengthen our bond with our partner and deepen intimacy when we forsake pillow talk for individually staring at our phones or tablets in bed? In the words of renowned couples' therapist, Esther Perel, "The last thing they [bedpartners] stroke is their phone. The first thing they stroke is their phone." But I digress. Back to the history lesson; I'll return to this important topic later in the book.

Around the eighteenth century, shared sleep began to be viewed negatively, at least among the upper class, and particularly among the aristocrats. This shift in attitudes coincided with an increase in the number of rooms in households of the time, which offered greater opportunities for privacy. Male aristocrats especially had a heightened sense of importance. Clergymen of all stripes began to view bedmates, especially if not limited to husband and wife, as immoral.

By the Victorian era (1837–1901) we began to see an even greater shift in cultural attitudes to value solitary sleep over shared sleep, at least for those who could afford it. Victorian sensibilities, with a heightened awareness of what it meant to be civilized, equated health with cleanliness, both day and night. Strict social codes that equated morality with privacy in the bedchamber contributed to a shift toward single beds among the wealthy. Half-baked science from the time also played a role. For example, the miasma theory held that disease was spread through poisonous particles in the air and could be identified by foul smells. Ergo, inhaling a partner's morning breath (or other bodily stinks) could literally make you sick, so best to sleep apart. In 1861 an influential doctor, William Whitty, offered the following sleep advice in his book *Sleep: Or the Hygiene of the Night*, "[People] should have a single bed in a large, clean, light, room, so as to pass all the hours of sleep in a pure fresh air, and that those who fail in this, will in the end fail in health and strength of limb and brain, and will die while yet their days are not all told." Wow. That's one scary public service announcement.

As is often the case, what began as a practice reserved for the rich soon began to take hold even among the less privileged. The middle class in many Western societies began viewing separate sleeping arrangements as an indicator of wealth and prestige, as well as moral superiority. Hence the proliferation of twin beds. In 1892 the *Yorkshire Herald* proclaimed, somewhat prophetically, "The twin-bed seems to have come to stay and will no doubt in time succeed the double bed in all rooms occupied by two persons." Although twin beds were not the norm per se, separate sleeping arrangements were generally seen as the healthier and, most importantly, the more socially acceptable option, spanning nearly a century into the 1950s.

Partly driving the allure of the twin bed was the somewhat puritanical and prudish morality adopted by the middle class, in reaction to the perceived debauchery and moral failings of the working classes and aristocracy. The twin bed was a symbol of purity and moral correctness, whereas the double bed was like a glaring advertisement for sex. Just think of the separate sleeping arrangements of Lucy and Ricky Ricardo on the TV show *I Love Lucy*. Although the actors were married in real life, each week the show featured the happy couple's nightly ritual of sleeping in separate twin beds.

Rules governing what was morally acceptable or unacceptable in film were spelled out under the Hays Code, named after William H. Hays, a devout Presbyterian and former postmaster general who was president of the Motion Pictures Producers and Distributors of America. The Hays code required at least one person to have their foot on the floor during any scene in which a couple was in a shared bed together. I guess the foot acted as some sort of chastity belt, ensuring the viewing audience that if any untoward behavior might occur, at least one of the parties could flee at a moment's notice. Compliance with the Hays Code persisted until the late 1960s.

But cultural attitudes about sex and the meaning of the marital bed started to shift back in the other direction earlier than that, coinciding with the sexual revolution. Twin beds began to be viewed by baby boomers as a relic of their parents' generation. Sex became increasingly recognized as a vital part of healthy unions. We began to equate the biblical meaning of sleeping together (i.e., sex) with the literal meaning, resulting in cultural attitudes that we still hold today: that sleeping apart is necessarily a sign of a loveless or sexless union. Only recently are we beginning to see another shift, where we are perhaps softening these rigid perceptions and opening the door to a more nuanced view of couples' sleeping arrangements—different strokes for different folks.

For many reasons, including greater independence within relationships and an aging population that faces more sleep problems (resulting in part from expanding waistlines, which can increase that probability), we are beginning to see the pendulum shift yet again today, with more couples—even those who are happily partnered—choosing to have separate bedrooms. Or perhaps they're just more willing to admit it. In 2007, the National Association of Homebuilders projected that by the year 2015, 60 percent of high-end custom homes would have dual main bedrooms. Obviously, 2015 has passed, and I haven't seen any more recent reports as to whether their projections came true, but nevertheless, as in the past, sleeping apart might be emerging as a privilege for those who can afford it. Despite these real estate trends and increasing media reports of everyday happy couples and celebrity couples, ranging from Rob Lowe and his wife, Sheryl Berkoff, to Donald and Melania Trump who, according to media reports, choose to sleep apart, there is still stigma. All these societal shifts back and forth across the continuum of sleeping together or sleeping apart have traditionally been based on little more than whims—half-baked ideas about what is right and what is wrong with little real evidence to back up those beliefs.

THE SCIENCE OF SHARED SLEEP

So what does the science actually tell us about the costs and benefits of sleeping together or apart? According to several studies, when sleep is measured objectively—particularly using wrist-worn devices called actigraphs that measure movement during sleep—people generally sleep worse with a partner. Early on in my career, I had the opportunity to meet with Dr. Robert Meadows, a sociologist from the University of Surrey, who was doing some fascinating work on the shared nature of sleep. In one study, in which he measured couples' sleep using actigraphy, he and his colleagues showed that "one-third of the variance in sleep is accounted for at the couple level." In other words, when looking at an individual's sleep pattern through the night, 30 percent of that individual's sleep (or lack thereof) is influenced by the bed partner's sleep. And in Meadow's words, "You can no longer ignore the impact of the bedpartner on one's sleep. Interdependence may be the defining feature of relationships, and in societies where it is common for adults to share a bed, it is also perhaps the defining feature of sleep."

Sharing a bed can be particularly detrimental to the bed partner's sleep if the other partner is a snorer—as you can likely imagine. In fact, if you sleep with a snorer, you can blame your partner for up to 50 percent of sleep disruptions. Given that men are more likely to be snorers than women, this may also be why several studies have also shown that women's sleep is more disturbed than men's when men and women share a bed.

Looking at this research alone, you might assume the science recommends we sleep apart, but a more recent study suggests sleeping together might be good for our sleep. A team of European researchers evaluated sleep in couples while sleeping with their partner versus sleeping apart. These researchers measured sleep using polysomnography, rather than actigraphy, as in much of the prior work on this topic. Polysomnography, or PSG, measures brain activity, muscle movements, eye movements, respiration, and heart rate during sleep and can capture sleep architecture or the different stages of sleep, including rapid eye movement sleep (REM), which is the type of sleep when dreams are most likely to occur. The researchers found that on nights when couples slept together, they showed a 10 percent increase in REM sleep, which may have benefits, as REM sleep is associated with memory consolidation and emotional processing.

On top of that, when you ask people, "Do you prefer to sleep with your partner, or do you prefer to sleep alone?," most will say they prefer to sleep with their partner, even if objective measures of their sleep show partner-derived disruption. As Dr. Meadows reflected to me, "The shared bed is a battleground. There's this really interesting tension we found as we started to identify novel forms of sleep disruption that were caused by the bed partner, but at the same time, people seemed to have a preference for sleeping with a partner." Stated simply, for many, the psychological benefits of cozying up to a trusted other outweigh the objective costs of sharing a bed. For at least some of us, our social brain is prioritizing our need for closeness and security at night even if it comes at a cost to our sleep.

In short, the answer to the million-dollar question "Do couples sleep better together or apart?" is: it depends. It depends on how sleep is measured, and it depends on the couple. There is no one-size-fits-all sleeping strategy for couples. But all couples should make sleep a priority because healthy sleep has the power to strengthen our relationships, whereas sleepless nights can bring relationship strife.

Rather than look for some sort of prescription for what couples should be doing, which, as we've seen through this tour through the history of the shared bed, is known to shift back and forth over time, I want you and your partner to focus on what you can do to maximize sleep quality for both of you. The key step is to use healthy and honest communication to find solutions that work for you as a couple, meeting the needs of both of you for sleep and for closeness and intimacy. If sleeping apart seems like the right choice for you as a couple, see it not as a failure in your relationship but as a commitment to making it stronger. Forge a sleep alliance with your partner based not on what society says you should do but on what gets you and your partner the best sleep you both need and deserve.

SHARED SLEEP ACTION PLAN:
Coupled Sleep Self-Assessment

As you work through this book, I'm going to ask that you and your partner complete a series of activities together. The goal of doing these activities is for you to come to a shared understanding and commitment for how you intend to spend that one-third of your lives together that happens while you're sleeping (or trying to sleep). This is your shared sleep action plan.

In this chapter, I explored how beliefs and expectations about the shared nature of sleep have changed throughout the ages. These fluctuations in attitudes about what is right and proper when it comes to couples and their sleeping arrangements helps illustrate just how silly it is to allow society to decide for us what we do in our own homes (and especially in our bedrooms) and within our own relationships. What matters most is what you and your partner expect, what you and your partner value, and what you and your partner need. In upcoming chapters, I'll explore just how important it is that you both get the rest your minds and bodies and your relationships need. Before I do, though, it's important that you both take some time to simply reflect on what you want in terms of sleep and why.

For this first step of your shared sleep action plan, you will interview each other. Follow the instructions for scoring the assessment, and then compare your answers and final results. My hope is that this provides the first spark of a discussion between you and your partner about how you as a couple want to manage this critical part of your relationship together.

I acknowledge this is not a scientifically validated instrument, and the exercises created for this book are not intended to be treatments. Rather, they are meant to help promote reflection and dialogue, and I hope they are fun activities to complete together (perhaps in bed). I encourage you to have an open mind about this exercise and your partner's responses. This is about learning more about each other, without judgment.

COUPLED SLEEP SELF-ASSESSMENT QUESTIONNAIRE

Question 1	How much sleep do you average each night?	Partner 1	Partner 2
A	Between 7 and 9 hours		
B	Between 6 and 7 hours		
C	Less than 6 hours or more than 9 hours*		
Question 2	How do you feel about your current sleeping arrangements?	Partner 1	Partner 2
A	Bedded bliss		
B	Okay		
C	Annoyed and unhappy		
Question 3	How important is it to you that you get healthy sleep?	Partner 1	Partner 2
A	Very important		
B	Somewhat important		
C	Not important		
Question 4	Do you feel you and your partner are on the same page when it comes to what you each need or want from your sleeping arrangement?	Partner 1	Partner 2
A	Yes		
B	Somewhat		
C	Not at all		
Question 5	How open are you to exploring changes to your sleeping arrangements?	Partner 1	Partner 2
A	I don't want to change		
B	I'd consider it		
C	I welcome it		

continues

To calculate your score, give yourself 1 point for each of your As, 2 points for each B, and 3 points for each C. Find your individual results below, and then compare those results with your partner's. Then, talk about it!

5–7: Snug as a bug. Your answers suggest that, for the most part, you are getting the sleep you want, you recognize the importance of sleep, and you like how things are working right now. If your partner has the same answers, you can read this book as a validation of what you seem to be doing well already (and regift it during the holidays). Look for couples who are clearly tired. They're not hard to find. They're everywhere!

8–11: Tossy turny. Your answers suggest that, while things aren't terrible, you aren't really getting what you want from your sleep and sleeping arrangements. Have you ever discussed this feeling with your partner? There's no time like the present.

9–15: Something must change. Your answers suggest you are very frustrated with your sleep and your sleeping situation with your partner, and sleep is low on the list of your priorities. Your ability to get enough sleep is important not only for your health but also for the health of your bond, so maybe it's time to shift some of those attitudes about sleep—if not for yourself, then for your partner.

* The evidence suggests that most adults need somewhere around seven to nine hours of sleep per night, which is considered optimal. Studies have shown that there may be health consequences for those who are "short" sleepers (less than seven hours) or "long" sleepers (more than nine hours), but there is variability across individuals in terms of sleep need. For example, if you are a competitive athlete, you may need more than the usual seven to nine hours of sleep, so don't sweat that. On the other hand, if you are someone who thinks that you are fine with sleeping less than six hours per night, consider this: only about 2 percent of the population are "natural short sleepers," meaning they can get away with sleeping less than the recommended sleep duration. So maybe you fall into that 2 percent, but statistically speaking you probably need more sleep.

PILLOW TALK PRIMERS

Now that you've both taken the Coupled Sleep Self-Assessment, consider cozying up in bed to explore one or more of the following questions together. If none of these questions works for you, feel free to think up your own, or even practice by sharing with your partner a recent dream you had. One study published in 2019 found that couples who talked about their dreams had higher levels of empathy, a key skill for fostering healthy relationships.

1. What was your best, worst, or weirdest night of sleep as a couple?
2. What are your beliefs about the importance of sleeping in the same bed together? Where do those beliefs come from? How do other influential relationships in your life (parents, grandparents, friends, etc.) manage their sleep routines?
3. What do the results of the sleep assessment tell you about your and your partner's feelings about the current state of things in your shared bed? What surprised you about the differences in your results, if any?
4. What do you want less or more of as it relates to your sleep or your sleeping situation?
5. How open are you to experimenting with making changes to your and your partner's sleep routine or arrangements? What experiments are you willing to try?
6. How does your sleep (or lack thereof) affect your ability to be the partner you want to be?

chapter two

SLEEP AS IF YOUR RELATIONSHIP DEPENDS ON IT

C HRIS WALKED INTO MY OFFICE, CASUALLY DRESSED, FRIENDLY, athletic-looking, and confident. I opened our initial session the way I typically do.

"Tell me about your sleep problems in your own words."

He gave a little groan, then said, "Honestly, I don't even know how to describe my sleep because it doesn't feel like I'm ever actually sleeping. Like a deep sleep. The thing is, I've got a lot to be grateful for in my life. I've got a good job, a wonderful wife, and three kids. I should be happy. I *should* be grateful. But I just can't. I'm too tired to feel any of those good things. It's like my brain is so focused on my sleep—I can't fit anything else in. What happens if I don't sleep again tonight? Will I be able to think clearly at my job? And what about once I get home? I literally don't have the mental capacity to deal with my family. I used to be the fun dad. You know, the one at the pool who throws all the kids up in the air, not just my own kids. But now, I'm just 'grumpy Dad.' And I know I'm not the husband I used to be. To be honest, I'm surprised Elizabeth keeps me around, I'm so not fun anymore. I have to spend every ounce of remaining energy I have just to put on a good face for work, but then I get home, and I just kind of give up. It's like I've got this hundred-pound gorilla weighing me down, and my family loses out the most."

Notice that when I asked Chris about his sleep problem, he quickly turned to the daytime consequences. That makes sense because insomnia, which was clearly plaguing him, is a twenty-four-hour disorder with the real distress often coming from the daytime ill effects rather than the sleep problem itself. Also, although he mentioned concern about the impact of his sleep problem on his work, he acknowledged that the interpersonal consequences, and his relationship with his wife specifically, were taking the biggest toll. As Chris was experiencing firsthand, sleep problems can jeopardize the very relationship we look to for security and comfort if they aren't addressed.

There are many ways that sleep problems can set you on a path toward a rocky relationship. Being in a good mood (most of the time) and reining in some of your bad moods or irritability, making sound decisions, problem solving, communicating effectively, tolerating frustration, practicing empathy: these are all important skills for cultivating and maintaining a healthy relationship. And these are also all the things that go south when you're low on sleep. When these are in short supply, whom do you take it out on? That's right: usually your partner.

Sleep loss is a profound mental and physical stressor, which makes it exceedingly difficult to be a supportive, engaged, loving, happy, or communicative partner. When our bodies are under stress, we are hardwired to respond in stereotyped ways, commonly known as the fight-or-flight response. This response primes our bodies and brains to deal with a real or imagined threat and leaves us with two primary options: to attack or retreat. From an evolutionary perspective, such responses serve a crucially important goal—to protect our survival. From a relationship perspective, however, this restricted response set comes at a major cost, heightening relationship tensions and even foretelling relationship demise.

We like to think of ourselves and our relationships as unique snowflakes. While there is some truth to that, in that every relationship has its own idiosyncrasies and every couple has their own set of experiences and personalities that are brought to bear on the relationship, some truisms can be applied to most relationships.

The renowned relationship expert and psychologist John Gottman has spent his career trying to crack the code of what makes some relationships succeed and others fail. While neither he nor other relationship researchers have developed prediction models with anywhere near 100 percent accuracy (if only), his work has shed light on some key characteristics that are harbingers of relationship doom. Gottman and colleagues identified four communication styles most predictive of relationship rupture, which they dub the Four Horsemen of the Apocalypse: criticism, contempt, defensiveness, and stonewalling. As shown in Figure 1, you can think of these "horsemen" along dimensions of attack or retreat, with criticism and contempt falling under the former, defensiveness and stonewalling falling under the latter. It's worth noting that "retreat," in this sense, is more aptly named "hostile retreat" to denote the negative style in which this type of withdrawing is conducted. There are, in fact, positive or healthy styles of retreat, such as telling your partner, "I know that this is a really important issue for us, but I need for us to table this conversation until tomorrow when I am less exhausted and more able to think and talk clearly." Hostile retreat, in contrast, goes something like this: "Whatever. I can't even deal with you!" or "Here we go again. Why should I even bother? It's not like you ever actually listen to what I'm saying." Eye rolling and sarcasm often go hand in hand with such quips. This kind of hostile retreat generally sends the message to your partner that you (a) don't care or (b) are oblivious to your partner's feelings or your role in the situation, both of which can be harmful to your relationship.

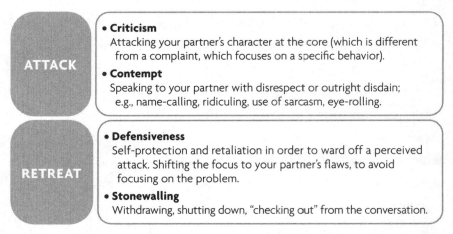

FIGURE 1. Four Horsemen of the Apocalypse in Relationships. Adapted from Dr. John Gottman, *The Seven Principles of Making Marriage Work.*

Sleep loss can set us on a path toward these polarized and equally toxic communication styles. The good news, however, is that for each of these toxic patterns, there is an antidote. The ability to use techniques like empathic understanding, active listening, use of "I" statements, and more, helps strengthen relationships. These skills are also easier to master when you're getting enough sleep. Chronic sleep loss or otherwise disturbed sleep, however, can trigger a host of emotions that can send you on a spiral of relationship-damaging behaviors.

YOU'RE JUST NOT NICE WHEN YOU'RE SLEEP-DEPRIVED

Jessica, a stay-at-home mom with a husband, Tim, who traveled regularly for work, and two children, five-year-old Benjamin and seven-year-old Penny, described to me how her sleep problems were getting in the way of her ability to cope with the everyday demands of family life. "When I am not sleeping well, it's like my emotions are in a state of hyper-electricity and there is static everywhere. They are like these frayed wires waiting to spark at the littlest thing. I lose my s**t over the littlest things. Kids are supposed to be loud and silly. They're supposed to make messes and have a hard time following directions. And Tim should be able to expect a wife who's happy to see him when he gets back from a long trip, but I just have no time for all that when I'm tired. And I'm always tired." I think we can all relate. And likely, if you ask your partner, they can too.

Most of us can immediately see the interpersonal consequences of sleep loss just by observing a toddler who has missed a nap. A normally easygoing, happy-go-lucky child can turn into an absolute terror—an irrational and emotional wreck (kicking, screaming, crying) after missing just one nap or if, God forbid, bedtime is delayed by an hour. While the symptoms of sleep loss are generally not quite so pronounced in adults, the truth is, as much as we try to fool ourselves into believing that we can get by while skimping on sleep, our emotions take a big hit, and so do our relationships.

Sleep plays a powerful role in how we experience and regulate our emotions. When we miss out on sleep, we become more irritable, we have more negative moods, our frustration tolerance is lowered, and we become more emotionally labile, meaning that we are more prone to mood swings, because our capacity to regulate our emotions is impaired.

Studies have shown that when sleep was restricted to five hours per night for a week, participants showed a progressive increase in negative emotions (e.g., anger, sadness, frustration, irritability), with each successive night of sleep restriction. Research has further shown that sleep loss led not only to increases in negative emotion but also decreases in positive emotion. To the partner of the person deprived of sleep, this activation of negative emotions in concert with the blunting of positive emotions can feel like a double whammy of contempt and criticism that's aggravated by being stonewalled. All in all, the partner feels lonely, vulnerable, and attacked, which, of course, can then lead to defensiveness or counterattack. Not a great recipe for relationship bliss.

Sleep loss not only makes us more unpleasant to be around but can also make us more susceptible to chronic mental illness. Sleep disturbances are a symptom of virtually every known mental health condition, and they exacerbate existing ones. They also can predict the onset of new mental health issues, including depression, anxiety, and even suicide. Left untreated, sleep problems predict poorer treatment response even to the most effective depression treatments and greater likelihood of depression relapse. They say depression hurts, and it does. But the hurt extends beyond the individual suffering from depression to the people closest to them. For example, a multinational study showed that depression increases the risk of divorce by about 60 percent. Prioritizing sleep and treating sleep problems is thus critical to supporting our mental health and, in doing so, supporting our relationship health as well.

Findings from brain imaging studies are starting to provide strong clues as to why sleep is so critically tied with our daily moods and our overall mental health. Under sleep-deprived conditions, people show increased activity in the amygdala, the emotion center of the brain, which can make us more emotionally reactive. At the same time, sleep-deprived brains show a dampening of response in the prefrontal cortical area, which is the part of the brain that controls the higher-order, executive functioning tasks. This is the part of the brain that might rein in the impulsive, emotionally reactive tendencies of the amygdala, but while sleep-deprived, it just doesn't do the job as well. The more sleep-deprived we become, the less aware we are of how sleep loss has impaired our emotions and behavior—this is a toxic combination. It's similar to the drunk guy in a bar stumbling around looking for his keys while insisting that he is perfectly fine. A sleep-deprived brain, similar to an inebriated brain, loses the ability to even recognize how impaired it is. Unfortunately, once we are in that sleep-induced, emotionally rattled state, this can set off a fuse, leading to increased likelihood of conflict and, most importantly, an increased likelihood of behaving badly once in conflict. You're like a powder keg waiting to explode.

BEWARE: EXPLOSIVE

Decades of relationship research has confirmed that conflict itself is not necessarily a sign of relationship doom or distress, as it is perfectly normal and in fact healthy to have some level of conflict in relationships. It's about how you engage in conflict with your partner that matters.

Social psychologists Drs. Amie Gordon and Serena Chen have studied couples' nightly sleep patterns and their daily relationship behaviors. They found that on nights when couples slept worse, they reported more conflict the next day. But it's not just that sleep loss increases the likelihood of conflict. It's that once a couple is in conflict, sleep loss triggers the very relationship behaviors and communication styles that we know are most toxic to relationships. As Dr. Gordon explains it, "When one or both partners are not well-rested, minor squabbles can turn into major rifts."

Researchers at the Ohio State University brought forty-three couples into the lab and asked them to engage in a typical relationship conflict. (It turns out that couples are very good at diving right into conflict when instructed to do so, even under the conspicuous conditions of a scientific laboratory, replete with a video camera to record the event.) Couples also reported on their nightly sleep patterns. After each conflict, the researchers painstakingly coded the conversation using a well-developed relationship coding system that identifies positive versus negative communication styles, including the degree of hostility or constructive responses. While all couples engaged in conflict, the researchers saw a clear distinction in *how* they engaged. Couples who reported sleeping less than seven hours per night were more likely to engage in hostile conflict. It's the difference between saying to your partner "It really makes me mad that you didn't unload the dishwasher" versus "Shocker—yet again, you couldn't do the one thing I asked you to do." The former statement is absolutely expressing disappointment, but it's specific, it focuses on how it makes the speaker feel, and it's not overly damning of the partner's overall character. On the other hand, the latter, hostile statement is laced with sarcasm and blame and generalizes to the partner's overall behaviors ("yet again"). The problem is that when one partner slams the other with a hostile remark, the receiving partner often feels as if they have no choice but to respond by attacking or retreating. You can see how sleep loss, even in just one partner, can have a domino effect on the other, leading to a nasty cycle, where neither partner is acting particularly nicely.

YOU JUST DON'T GET ME

A sure-fire way to ratchet up the intensity of a relationship tiff is when one or both partners feel their words and, more importantly, their feelings are not being heard. In many ways, empathy is the glue that binds a relationship together. Author, public speaker, and professor of social work Brené Brown describes empathy as "simply listening, holding space, withholding judgment, emotionally connecting, and communicating that incredibly healing message of you're not alone." A sense of mutual empathy is a fundamental characteristic of a secure relationship.

While we often think that empathy equates to expressions like "I know what you're feeling," research suggests that genuine expressions of empathy are rooted in the ability to read another person's emotions and put one's self in another person's shoes. This is called "empathic accuracy." While it is certainly true that you cannot be expected to read your partner's mind, being able to gauge your partner's emotional temperature during a hot-topic discussion is a critically important skill for relationship well-being. Sometimes the best thing you can do as a partner is to gently back off when you recognize that emotions are just a bit too raw. Fail to miss those cues, and you run the risk of being the proverbial bull in a china shop—coming on way too strong when your partner is already feeling vulnerable. Unfortunately, empathic accuracy also takes a hit when relationship partners are sleep-deprived.

Drs. Gordon and Chen found not only that couples were more likely to engage in conflict after sleeping poorly but also that poorly slept people had lower empathic accuracy. Their research showed that the negative effects of one partner's sleep loss on empathic accuracy spread to the other partner. On nights when one partner slept worse, the other partner also showed reductions in empathic accuracy. This likely reflects a relationship dynamic in which one partner feels dismissed or that their feelings aren't being heard, leading to increased defensiveness and emotional walls being built up on both sides.

CAN WE TALK?

Other research shows that even the words we use to communicate and the sounds of our voices are colored by our sleep or lack thereof. Psychologist Eleanor McGlinchey used computerized text analysis, including analysis of acoustic properties of speech, as well as observer ratings of the emotional expression of speech, before and after sleep deprivation in the laboratory. She wanted to determine the extent to which sleep deprivation affected word choice, including positive and negative emotion words, like "happy" or "excited" or "sad" or "anxious," as well as the tone, including positive and negative emotion expression. She found that under sleep-deprived conditions, participants showed a decrease in the use of positive emotion words. To investigate changes in vocal tone, she had trained observers (who were unaware of the participants' sleep conditions) listen to the speeches and rate the quality of the emotional expression of the speech, before and after the participants were sleep-deprived. When participants were sleep-deprived, observers rated the speech as being lower in positive emotional expression (less happy or calm) and higher in negative emotional expression (more sad, anxious, or fatigued).

Using sophisticated computerized text analysis of the acoustic properties of speech, she also found that sleep-deprived participants' speech was "softer, sharper, and lower energy," said McGlinchey. "In fact, this combination of vocal properties that we saw under sleep-deprived conditions is akin to what computerized text analysis has found for people who are standing trial in a courtroom. In other words, they sound stressed and defensive, and the lower acoustic energy can make it sound like the person is disengaged." Just think about this finding in the context of having a difficult argument with your partner. The vocal tone you are giving off when you are poorly slept sounds stressed, less happy, more sad, and less engaged—hardly a recipe for effective communication. And the thing of it is, you can't really control the acoustic properties of your voice. That just happens when you are sleep-deprived.

The words we use and the tone of our voice when communicating matters—especially in conflict. Industrial-organizational psychologists who study communication in corporate environments have identified that one of the keys to conflict resolution is creating a safe environment, characterized by mutual respect and mutual goals for the discussion to occur. In turn, mutual respect is conveyed by our tone of voice and the words and facial expressions we use. Sleep loss can cast a pall over our communication skills, increasing the likelihood of conflict escalation rather than finding a healthy way out, which requires good communication and good decision-making skills.

RISKY BUSINESS

We make decisions all the time that can help or hurt our relationships. From the relatively mundane decisions, such as, "Do I tell my husband now that I really don't want to spend Thanksgiving with his parents, or do I wait until a more opportune time?" to the bigger risk decisions like, "Do I respond to a flirtatious email from a colleague?" When we don't sleep enough or our sleep is disturbed, we just don't think clearly. Studies have shown that under sleep-deprived conditions, decision making is harder. We are more distracted and more prone to risky or impulsive behaviors, which can be harmful to our relationships. And despite our obsession with venti cappuccinos, energy drinks, and the like, studies have also shown that caffeine is no antidote to the compromised decision making that results from sleep deprivation. Researchers at Walter Reed Army Research Institute showed that sleep-deprived subjects who participated in a gambling task made much riskier decisions than their well-slept counterparts, and their decisions were just as bad after consuming four two-hundred-milligram doses of caffeine, which is about the equivalent of drinking four tall Starbucks coffees.

Not only do we make riskier decisions while sleep-deprived, but our moral compass is also askew. Those same researchers at Walter Reed presented subjects with a series of moral dilemmas and asked them to judge the appropriateness of various courses of action under rested and sleep-deprived conditions. Under sleep-deprived conditions, subjects took significantly longer to decide on a course of action, as compared to the rested condition. The researchers note that this doesn't imply that sleep loss makes you a "less moral" person, but it does tax your decision-making skills, making moral dilemmas (e.g., do you make the choice that benefits you or the broader good?) that much more challenging. Over time, if sleepless nights persist, this can chip away at your resolve, potentially leading to a ripple effect of seemingly harmless decisions (at least in isolation) that collectively can make a big and damaging splash in your relationship.

TWO CAN BE THE LONELIEST NUMBER

Beyond the sleep-induced relationship blowups and bad decisions caused by poor sleep, lack of sleep can lead to broader social consequences, including the more existential state of loneliness. Science tells us that social isolation and loneliness are not the same thing. You can be lonely even in a relationship, and it sure doesn't feel good to either partner.

New science is showing us that lack of sleep hurts our social brains and can make us feel alone in the world. In a series of elegant studies published in 2018, researchers at the University of California, Berkeley, found that poor sleep predicted greater feelings of loneliness, as well as greater social withdrawal and anxiety, the next day. At the brain level, the researchers demonstrated that sleep-deprived people showed deactivation in the parts of the brain that are responsible for helping understand other people's actions and behaviors, and amplification in the parts of the brain that signal threat or fear responses in social contexts. In other words, sleep-deprived subjects' brains were less active in the parts of the brain that make you more social and more active in the parts of the brain that make you want to stand in the corner away from people. The final piece of this research is perhaps even more fascinating because, in addition to looking at the brains and behaviors of these sleep-deprived subjects, they also looked at how other people reacted to the sleep-deprived subjects. They found that the observers perceived the sleep-deprived people to be lonelier and less attractive than well-slept people. But the real kicker is that after observing the people who were sleep-deprived, the observers themselves reported feeling lonelier and more socially withdrawn, despite being well-rested.

Sleep-induced loneliness, therefore, is contagious. Within couples, this can lead to greater emotional distancing and a lack of connection with your partner. I have seen the demise of many relationships for this very reason. These are the couples who break up or divorce, and everyone around them can't understand why the relationship didn't work out because there didn't seem to be any overt hostility or anger between the partners. But behind closed doors, they were living separate lives.

Take my client Susan, for example. She was a forty-eight-year-old woman who had been married for nine years to her husband Dave, and with whom she had three young children. "We were just two ships, passing by each other and giving each other lists of things to do, but not actually sharing any meaningful or positive connection with each other anymore," she said. "Since our third child was born [five years earlier], we've been living like this. And for all these years I have been telling myself all these excuses to stay, like it's worth it for the kids, or it's not really so bad because it's not like we are fighting all the time or anything. The problem is we just aren't partners anymore. But for the past two years, it's just gotten so hard, because I feel like there is this person in my home that I used to be in love with and connected to, and now our relationship is just a series of transactions. I feel no closer to him than I do the clerk in the grocery store, and yet we are living under the same roof. It's the loneliest I have ever felt, and it's unbearable. That's why I knew I had to end this. I know it won't be easy being a single mom, but at least I know I am alone by choice. Alone in a marriage feels far worse."

There were likely other factors than a lack of sleep that contributed to Susan's feelings of loneliness, but the research is clear: a lack of sleep for one or more partners fosters behaviors, moods, and emotional states that serve to create distance between couples. If allowed to persist for too long, that distance can create long term and potentially permanent damage to the relationship.

NOT TONIGHT, HONEY—I'M TOO TIRED

So far I've talked a lot about how sleep loss can set us up for greater emotional distancing and negative conflict tactics within relationships, but I would be remiss if I didn't also mention how sleep loss can negatively affect our physical connection and intimacy. According to sex researchers, "feeling too tired" is one of the most frequently heard excuses for skipping out on sex. While it may, for some, feel like no more than an excuse, there is some converging science to show that sleep loss can hurt our sex lives. For example, a University of Michigan study of women's sleep and sexual activity found that when women slept poorly they reported less sexual desire and less frequent sexual activity the next day.

And it's not just women's sex drive that's affected by sleep loss. A 2011 study published in the preeminent medical journal

Journal of the American Medical Association found that men who were restricted to five hours of sleep for eight consecutive nights had a 10 to 15 percent reduction in testosterone levels, which can have a big impact on sex drive. To put that into context, that level of decline in testosterone is about the equivalent of aging a man by ten to fifteen years. A more recent study showed a positive, linear relationship between sleep duration and testicular volume. In other words, the more sleep the men were getting, the larger the testes. Now we've all heard that size doesn't matter, but when it comes to male fertility, size actually does matter. There is a direct correlation between testes size and sperm count. So for couples looking to enhance their sex life as well as those seeking to expand their family, it's time to start prioritizing sleep.

MAKING AMENDS

Chris, my client whose story I shared at the start of this chapter, recognized that his sleep problems were having such a negative effect on him, his wife, and his entire family that he had to seek professional help. By using a combination of the sleep and relationship diaries I'll share with you at the end of this chapter, Chris began to see how his daily fluctuations in sleep affected his relationship behaviors. This wasn't an easy process. Chronicling how his sleep problems had been affecting his family and recognizing that this had been going on for months before he eventually sought treatment led to his feeling a lot of guilt. Unfortunately, guilt does not always produce the kind of behavior change we are looking for. Instead, guilt can make us feel paralyzed, unworthy, and incapable of change. Becoming more aware of how his sleep problems influenced his behavior allowed him some healthy distance to be able to recognize that he wasn't a fundamentally flawed person, but that he couldn't be the person he wanted to be for his family when not sleeping well.

From there he could take personal responsibility for his actions. He made amends with his wife for neglecting her needs and for not being the partner she needed him to be for the many months when his sleep problems went untreated. In addition to his heartfelt apology, he consciously changed his behavior. The latter involved taking a more active role in the family and engaging in strategies to increase his energy levels after work, like taking a walk with the kids as they rode their bikes as soon as he got home. Most importantly, he stuck with treatment (Cognitive Behavioral Therapy for Insomnia) even when it was tough. As a result, his sleep improved. He and his family reaped the benefits.

"I have my husband back," Chris's wife, Elizabeth, told me when they both came in for his final session. "It's like he's actually present and making an effort to be a part of the family now."

As a sleep clinician, it's especially rewarding for me when I get to witness the spillover benefits of effective sleep treatment on my patient as well as his family. It's these very benefits I hope you, your partner, and your family can receive from your efforts to get more and better sleep in your life.

SHARED SLEEP ACTION PLAN:
Logging Your Sleep Together

As you reach the end of this chapter, you may be entering a state of increasing anxiety, verging on panic for some, as I describe the litany of relationship harms that could be caused by sleep loss. And if that isn't frightening enough, in the next chapter I'll discuss how a vicious cycle between poor sleep and poor relationships can trigger a toxic dance that also threatens your physical and mental health. Frankly, the last thing any of us needs is yet another reason to keep us up at night. Don't fret. There is hope. Rather than sweating the consequences of sleep loss, it's time to start prioritizing sleep as a mutual goal within your relationship. Here are some simple strategies to get you started on a path to personal awareness of how sleep affects your relationship and what you can do about it.

For this part of your Shared Sleep Action Plan, I want you and your partner to complete a sleep diary and a relationship diary. The goal for these two diaries is for you both to begin to recognize how your sleep and relationship quality varies day to day so you can start to identify interconnections between them. My research has shown that sleep loss affects relationships and relationship issues affect our ability to sleep. These diaries can help you fully understand and appreciate this bidirectional nature of the shared sleep experience.

The diaries are your own; they should be kept confidential. But if you and your partner both complete diaries, which I encourage you to do, feel free to discuss your findings with each other after. Do you see any patterns emerging? On nights when you slept better or longer, how did you rate your relationship quality the next day? On days when you had a conflict with your spouse (not to worry, we all have them), was there any impact on your sleep? This is your opportunity to do your own investigation: to identify the pathways and the opportunities for you and your partner to improve your sleep and relationship quality. Of course, if you identify sleep or relationship issues that are beyond your ability to manage, this is also a great opportunity to recognize that you may need professional help from a sleep or relationship specialist. There is no shame in that! In fact, that's exactly what my client Chris did.

The Sleep Diary

One of the first steps for any behavioral change is to start logging the behavior you wish to change. That's why fitness trackers and diet apps are big business these days. For my clients, I generally find it most useful to go the low-tech route and start by writing down the behaviors you are trying to change. Every morning upon awakening, record your bedtimes and wake-up times from the previous night and your subjective sleep quality on a scale of 1 to 10 (you'll find an example at the end of this chapter). Don't worry about accuracy, at least in terms of what the clock says. In fact, don't look at the clock at all once you go to sleep. Nothing good ever comes from finding out what time it is if you wake up in the middle of the night. Just give your best guess of when you went to bed and when you woke up in the morning. That will be close enough.

SLEEP DIARY

DAY'S DATE	8/10/20	DATE
What time did you get to bed?	10:00 p.m.	
What did you do in bed before falling asleep? (e.g., Watch tv, have sex, read a book, read emails, etc.)	Watch TV with my spouse	
What time did you actually try to fall asleep (i.e., Lights out)	10:30 p.m.	
How long do you think it took to fall asleep?	10 minutes	
How many times did you wake up in the night, not including your final awakening?	Twice	
How long in total did all of your middle of the night awakenings last?	<30 minutes	
What was the main reason(s) for your middle of the night awakenings? (e.g. No particular reason, go to the bathroom, child, partner snoring)	Teenager came home late; had to go to the bathroom	
What time was your final awakening?	5:55 a.m	
What time did you get out of bed for the day?	6:00 a.m.	
How would you rate your sleep quality? (1–10 scale with 1 = Very Bad and 10 = Excellent)	8	
Did you sleep with your partner last night?	Yes	

DATE	DATE	DATE	DATE	DATE	DATE

The Relationship Diary

Every evening, fill out the relationship diary. (You'll want to make enough copies of the blank version for however many days you plan to record.) Keeping this diary will tap into several key aspects of relationship functioning, ranging from how much you felt supported or valued by your spouse to how much conflict you had with your spouse that day. Remember, conflict itself is not the problem. It's how you and your partner engaged in the conflict. The relationship diary is a great opportunity to notice variability in the quality of your relationship day to day. After all, we all have our relationship ups and downs. But if you notice that your relationship is weighted on the "down" side, now is the chance to do something about it, including prioritizing your sleep.

RELATIONSHIP DIARY

Instructions for filling out the daily relationship diary:

1. Fill out the relationship diary at the end of the day, but at least one hour before bedtime.

2. Diaries should be filled out independently of your partner.

3. Use an "X" mark on the line below to indicate how much you felt each of the items or if you prefer you can use a numeric scale from 1–10 with one being very little up to 10 being very much.

During today's interaction with your spouse to what extent did you feel . . .	
1. Supported?	Very Little _____ Very Much
2. Criticized?	Very Little _____ Very Much
3. Close to your spouse?	Very Little _____ Very Much
4. Dismissed?	Very Little _____ Very Much
5. Ignored?	Very Little _____ Very Much
6. Valued by your spouse?	Very Little _____ Very Much
7. Did you discuss personal feelings with your spouse?	Very Little _____ Very Much
8. Did you and your spouse do any pleasurable activities together?	Very Little _____ Very Much
9. Did you and your spouse argue/have a conflict?	Very Little _____ Very Much
10. If yes, think of the most intense conflict, how severe was it?	Minor Tiff _____ Major Blow-up

chapter three

A TOXIC DANCE

THE DOWNWARD SPIRAL FOR STEPHEN AND NICOLE BEGAN AFTER they experienced a health scare with their infant son that rocked their relationship to its core. Stephen was taking care of seven-month-old Ben while Nicole was out for a run. Stephen was going to take Ben to the park, so he had placed him in his little bucket car seat on the kitchen table, as he had done hundreds of times before. Ben wasn't buckled into his seat yet. For the briefest instant, Stephen turned to grab his keys, which were lying on the counter. Then he heard a *thunk*. Stephen spun around, and for a terrifying moment, there was silence, with Ben unmoving on the floor and the car seat flipped partially on top of him. "That was honestly the scariest part of all. Seeing Ben lying there but not making a sound. Then he started to wail. It was awful, but in a way a relief—just to know he was doing what a kid should do when he gets hurt and not just knocked out."

Stephen grabbed Ben and jumped into the car to take him to the children's hospital. He called Nicole on his way and told her to meet him there. She arrived at the emergency room soon after Stephen and Ben. Together they waited to see the doctor, who immediately ordered a CT scan. The biggest concern was whether Ben experienced significant head trauma. As they waited for the scan results, Stephen was a "total basket case," replaying in his head what he must have done wrong. Nicole was shaken herself, but she knew Stephen needed her strength and support. She hugged him and told him that "it wasn't his fault" and that "freaky accidents happen with babies."

Thankfully, the scan results showed no signs of brain trauma, which was a huge relief to both Stephen and Nicole. But as their doctor informed them, many forms of traumatic brain injury will not show up on a scan. So they were sent home with the recommendation to pay close attention to Ben's behavior, including excessive sleepiness, inconsolable crying, refusal to sleep, loss of consciousness, or vomiting. Walking out of the hospital that day, both Stephen and Nicole were speechless and in a state of terror, feeling as if they might have dodged a bullet, but not being totally in the clear. As first-time parents, they felt crushed by the weight of this terror.

In the weeks that followed, they watched Ben like hawks for any signs of brain trauma, which, fortunately, did not appear. In those initial weeks, when they were both hypervigilant and entirely focused on observing Ben, watching and waiting for a sign that something was really wrong with their baby's brain, they had a sort of solidarity in their shared vigilance. Ironically, though, as the weeks passed, and it became clearer that Ben was really okay, their relationship (and their sleep) started to take a turn for the worse.

In subtle (and sometimes not-too-subtle) ways, Stephen felt blamed, mistrusted, and questioned whenever he did anything with Ben, whether strapping him into the car seat or putting him to bed at night. Their relationship became strained, and both felt disconnected and alone. "I know it sounds dramatic," Stephen described, "but I think we both were feeling a bit of PTSD, even after we knew Ben was going to be fine."

Like anyone who has experienced a trauma, both Stephen and Nicole's sleep also suffered. Not only were they waking in the middle of the night, feeling the need to check on Ben even as he slept, but they were so on edge with each other throughout the day that lying in bed together just exacerbated their problems. "I felt like I was sleeping with the enemy," said Nicole. Strong negative emotions, including anger and hurt, invaded their bedroom, setting them up for many sleepless nights. Neither felt they could talk about their pain and fear because Stephen felt shamed and blamed and Nicole felt helpless, angry, and disconnected. And the sleep deprivation they were both experiencing certainly didn't help their communication skills or their ability to regulate their emotions. Over time, they started to resent each other, and sometimes neither could contain their contempt for the other, resulting in hurtful words and actions.

They both felt betrayed, because the most basic tenet of their relationship—that they would never intentionally hurt one another—had been violated. Stephen once told me that "in a way, if she had an affair, it might not have hurt so bad. But her turning on me like that, and blaming me for the accident, and holding it against me, like I was intentionally being a bad father, was the biggest betrayal of all." Ultimately, with time and really good individual and couple's therapy, they repaired their relationship, but it took several years to heal. "Honestly," said Nicole, "we were very close to divorce. We both had to undo years of damage to each other and find ways to forgive. It brought out the worst in us, to feel so vulnerable, and to not be able to count on each other anymore when we needed each other the most. It was our marital rock bottom. But I am glad we held on."

This kind of vicious, downward spiral between relationship strife and sleepless nights can strike couples of all ages and walks of life and for a variety of different causes. For some, it may be sleep disruption in one or both partners driving the vicious cycle and leading to relationship conflict and withdrawal. For others, like Stephen and Nicole, it can be a hit to the relationship that triggers a cascade of emotional and behavioral consequences, leading to disrupted sleep. Whatever the cause, because relationship quality and sleep go hand in hand, once the spiral starts, it can be very hard to get out of it. And this negative spiral can have far-reaching effects on our mental and physical health.

Many of us can think of situations in our own lives when intense stress has resulted in not being able to sleep. When that happens long enough, we can begin to feel like a walking petri dish—seemingly susceptible to every germ, virus, or bacteria that happens to be floating around. In fact, research has shown that sleep loss can compromise immune functioning and increase risk for viruses, such as the common cold—a particularly important reminder in the age of the COVID-19 pandemic, when sleep problems are aplenty, and it has never been more critical to promote healthy immune systems.

Just as good sleep is vital for health, so are good relationships. Science shows us, for instance, that happily married or partnered people have lower rates of depression and heart disease and live longer than those who are unmarried or unpartnered. Since sleep and the quality of our relationships are interconnected, when either or both go south, this can be a toxic two-step.

I experienced this phenomenon personally after the birth of my first child. Like every parent of a newborn, I was definitely sleep-deprived, and for the first time in our married life, my husband and I had a lot to fight over. And fight we did.

In retrospect, while they seemed significant at the time, our fights were nothing major—basically the usual anxious new-parent stuff—but our collective lack of sleep, the stress of being new parents, and both of our reactions to those issues amplified their significance and were taking a toll in a lot of ways, including on my health. For about the first six months of my son's life, I felt subclinically ill. It wasn't severe, but I had some sort of cold or virus the entire time. This was especially striking to me because I rarely get sick. It was more than just coincidence.

Science clearly demonstrates that both sleep and relationship quality can have an impact on our physical and mental health, and collectively, if they go awry, they can really do some damage. On the other hand, a high-quality relationship may buffer the adverse consequences of sleep disturbances, or conversely, maintaining healthy sleep in the context of relationship difficulties may mitigate the negative effects of problems in one's relationship.

In 2001, researchers from the Ohio State University published what is now a landmark review article, and one of the most influential articles on my professional career, entitled "Marriage and Health: His and Hers." The article summarized the existing scientific evidence concerning the health consequences of high-conflict (or otherwise unhappy) relationships, and they compared them with the health benefits of supportive and high-functioning relationships.

They also provided a framework for understanding the potential pathways, including increased risk of depression, poor health habits, and stress-related physiological mechanisms that could plausibly explain how something as seemingly unrelated as how you interact with your spouse could literally get under your skin to impact chronic health conditions like heart disease, diabetes, or even cancer. In the past two decades following the article's publication, the research has only grown, with more and more data to suggest that being in a happy marriage not only feels good but can literally make us live longer, happier, and healthier lives.

When I read this research in graduate school, I was fascinated by the idea that a miserable marriage could make you sick. In the early stages of my career, I published several studies in which we tried to "unpack" whether the benefits of marriage were due to simply "being married" (or having a partner) or if what really mattered was being in a high-quality marriage. This may sound like a "no duh" sort of question to just about anyone who has ever been in a relationship—I mean, of course the quality matters! But as scientists, it is sometimes our job to demonstrate what seems intrinsically obvious to just about everyone else and to investigate the underlying causes, which are often less obvious and sometimes even counterintuitive. And sure enough, what we and others have found is that being in a happy marriage does confer health benefits, including lowering risk for heart disease, but being in an unhappy marriage actually increases one's risk, even above being unpartnered. In other words, being in a committed relationship is good for one's health, but only if it is a happy one.

As obvious as these findings may seem to some, this set me on a path to try to better understand how the good parts of relationships actually manifest as being good for your health. This is why the

Ohio State review article I mentioned had such an impact on me: it comprehensively laid out for the first time all of the key pathways that might explain how good relationships make us feel good both inside and out and conversely how bad relationships can make us feel bad and literally make us sick. And as comprehensive as their review was, the thing that really struck me was what was missing. The missing piece was that crucial third of our lives that couples generally spend together and that is vitally important for health: sleep. Ultimately, this helped launch my career, which has, ever since, been focused on trying to understand how sleep and relationship quality are intertwined and how their interplay affects our health, our well-being, and even our survival.

My research and that of others have clearly shown how the quality of our sleep and our relationships can serve to work together to enhance our health and happiness or against each other to drag it down. In Chapter 2, I discussed how sleep loss can negatively impact relationship quality by undermining our ability to regulate emotions and our decision-making and communication skills, among other things. Research also shows us that the quality of our relationships can affect our sleep; this can give rise to a health-damaging or health-promoting feedback loop. For example, when we studied married, heterosexual couples' sleep and relationship quality over ten days, we found that men who slept worse reported worse relationship functioning the next day. We found evidence for the reverse direction in women. That is, when a woman reported less positive or more negative relationship functioning during the day, both her sleep *and* her husband's sleep suffered that night. As the saying goes, if she's not happy . . . no one's sleeping. (Just ask my husband.)

Multiple studies have shown the importance of a quality relationship for sleep. That quality is achieved when couples practice specific behaviors that typify strong relationships. When thinking about the qualities in a relationship that promote healthy sleep versus those that might lead to sleep disruption, it's important to harken back to that evolutionary framework I mentioned in Chapter 1. From an evolutionary standpoint, sleep is a vulnerable state to be in—you are lying down, semiconscious, eyes closed. In other words, easy prey for the wandering predator. That's where the presence and quality of our relationships play such an important role. Human beings are social beings. It is in our DNA to depend on our social connections to help us feel safe and secure and to support our survival. But not all relationships are created equal. While some relationships provide that feeling of warmth, protection, and security, which should facilitate healthy sleep by allowing one to dampen down vigilance and arousal, particularly at night, other relationships can actually amp up vigilance, by making one feel always on one's toes or backed against the wall. Such emotional and physiological arousal is antithetical to the ability to fall into deep, satisfying sleep. For example, research has shown that having a high level of attachment anxiety, a term used by relationship researchers to refer to a feeling of being preoccupied or worried about whether your partner will be there for you in times of need, is associated with poorer sleep quality and lesser objectively measured "deep sleep"—the type of sleep that is thought to promote restoration and other health benefits.

At the extreme end of this relationship dimension of vigilance, you can think of relationships characterized by high levels of toxic conflict (recall the Four Horsemen mentioned in Chapter 2) or even violence. It will likely come as no surprise to anyone that victims of domestic violence experience high levels of sleep problems, in part because violence in the home fosters a constant state of vigilance. Furthermore, even among victims who leave their abuser, sleep problems can be lasting, given that domestic violence often occurs at night and in the bedroom, creating a learned association between the bedroom and fear, which is hardly conducive to healthy sleep.

Even at lesser extremes of relationship problems, it is important to recognize and identify if there are aspects of your relationship that are tipping the scales toward fostering vigilance, and to intervene, including seeking professional help as necessary. Ask yourself some simple questions to see where you fall on that spectrum. For example: Do I feel safe in my relationship? Do I feel that my partner is there for me and will be there for me in times of need? Do I feel that my partner holds dear my best interests and well-being?

It is also critical to recognize and continue to develop those aspects of your relationship that help to foster feelings of safety and security that can benefit sleep as well as your overall health and well-being. One such behavior is the ability and willingness to be vulnerable and open as partners. Research has shown that couples who were able to share their personal thoughts and feelings with each other experience better sleep quality and more efficient sleep. This was true for men and for women. Another such behavior is practicing gratitude, which science has shown is good for relationships and good for sleep. Taking a few minutes at the end of the day to simply debrief with some pillow talk and express gratitude for each other might be yet another habit to develop to help bolster the quality of your shared sleep and your relationship.

It's important to understand how and why relationships get off course, just as it's important to understand how sleep loss can negatively affect our relationships and our health, because recognizing these downstream consequences is the first step to identifying opportunities for intervention and change. Science has given us some strong hints about how and why relationships can affect sleep and sleep can affect our relationships, and how this feedback loop can have an impact on our physical health. The remainder of this chapter unveils how relationship quality, sleep, and their interplay can have a powerful effect on our physical health, by influencing our mental health, our health-related behaviors, and our body's stress response system.

MENTAL HEALTH

In Chapter 2, I discussed the powerful role of sleep in influencing moods and how sleep disturbances can lead to an increased risk of developing mental health problems, including the most common mental health disorder, depression. Being in a healthy relationship is also beneficial for your mental health. People who are in healthy relationships experience more positive moods and fewer negative moods, have lower rates of depression, and are less likely to complete suicide than those who are in unhealthy relationships or unpartnered. The ritual of going to bed together, and holding that time together as sacred, may also buffer against intense negative emotions, counteracting the stresses of the day and reducing psychological and physiological arousal prior to falling asleep.

On the flip side, relationship problems are a potent source of stress, which can breed ruminative thoughts (the type of thoughts that appear to be on a loop, like a broken record). These incessant and intrusive thoughts, particularly when they occupy your brain at bedtime, can wreak havoc on sleep and mental health, especially if you are sleeping next to the object of your animosity.

Our mental health, in turn, is strongly linked with our physical health. The saying "depression hurts" is literally true. For instance, being depressed increases your risk of having a heart attack or stroke, and among heart attack survivors, being depressed doubles or triples the risk of mortality, compared to those without depression. As a result of these and other findings linking depression with both increased risk of heart attack and poorer prognosis following heart attack, depression has joined the ranks of other, established risk factors for heart disease including obesity, high blood pressure, and smoking. Both sleep and relationship problems can lead to clinically significant mental health problems, which not only hurts in the emotional sense but can also set you up for increased risk for physical health problems, including heart disease and early death.

BEHAVIOR

Relationships are health-protective because partners can motivate us to take better care of ourselves. Maybe your partner encourages you to get to the gym, take your medications, stop smoking, or eat a healthy diet. Scientists call this "social control." Partners often call it "nagging." But in its best light, social control can be an important way to increase the likelihood of engaging in positive health behaviors, such as getting sufficient exercise, eating a healthy diet, and getting good-quality sleep, and to deter against negative health behaviors, such as smoking, excessive alcohol use, drug use, or staying up into the wee hours while binge-watching Netflix or gaming. This type of influence by one's partner can be profoundly beneficial for one's health, and it is likely one of the reasons why partnered people live longer, happier, and healthier lives than their unpartnered counterparts.

When it comes to bedtime and healthy sleep behaviors, partners play an important role here too. For many couples, the shared act of going to bed at the same time is crucial to preserving a consistent bedtime routine. When talking with couples about why they prefer to sleep with a partner, an oft-repeated reason goes something like this: "If it weren't for my wife, my sleep schedule would go out the window. I'd just get sucked into watching TV or logging on to my computer into the wee hours of the morning. But she helps rein me in. And besides, once I pull myself away from the computer or TV, it's actually really nice to lie in bed next to her." Our research has shown that for a woman, after a night when she reports going to bed at the same time as her spouse, she reports better relationship quality the next day, suggesting that the shared ritual of going to bed with her partner may benefit their relationship.

Of course, it's not always possible for couples to go to bed at the same time. Maybe they have different work schedules, or maybe one is a morning lark and the other is a night owl. These different schedules can be challenging to negotiate. In these situations, it's critical that both individuals in the couple recognize that they each have competing needs, schedules, and sleep-wake preferences. Even so, preserving the ritual of at least spending some time together in bed, perhaps before one of them falls asleep, can help promote more consistent bedtime routines and can be an important opportunity to relax and connect with their partner.

A romantic partner can also have a direct impact on our sleep by influencing the regularity of our routines, including our sleep-wake behaviors. Scientists who study circadian rhythms use the German word *zeitgeber*, meaning "time keeper," to refer to the external cues that help to set our internal circadian rhythms to a roughly twenty-four-hour cycle. Although exposure to light is the most powerful zeitgeber (which is why exposure to light in the morning is important to cue alertness, and reducing light at bedtime is key to facilitating sleepiness), there are other zeitgebers that are more social in nature. For example, the timing of our first contact with a human being, as well as mealtimes and wake-up times, can help to set our internal circadian rhythms and in turn influence our sleep as well as our overall health and well-being. Because couples often engage in these behaviors together, and partners help to regulate when and if these behaviors occur, a rift in the relationship can cause a disruption to these health-promoting daily rhythms that are often synchronized within couples. And as partners' daily schedules diverge and partners live parallel lives, this can exacerbate feelings of isolation and disconnection, resulting in a cascade of consequences for the relationship, the couples' sleep, and potentially both partners' health.

STRESS RESPONSE

Stress comes in many forms, including relationship stress stemming from a conflict with a significant other, or perhaps it's more of an existential concern regarding whether your partner will really be there for you emotionally and physically in times of need. Stress can also arise from not sleeping well. In my clinical practice, I regularly see clients who are otherwise healthy and high functioning and would generally describe themselves as "not being much of a worrier about most things," but when it comes to sleep, "that's a major source" of stress and worry. Whether from the stress of a high-conflict relationship or from the stress of nightly battles with sleep, our brains and our bodies are hardwired to elicit what has been referred to as the fight-or-flight response. The fight-or-flight response involves a coordinated set of physiological responses, including activation of the central nervous system, that leads to increases in blood pressure, heart rate, and galvanic skin responses (for example, you sweat when stressed); release of stress hormones, such as cortisol; and suppression of the immune system and activation of the inflammatory response system. Heightened inflammatory responses, in turn, are thought to be involved in virtually all current major causes of morbidity and mortality, from heart disease to dementia.

In one of my favorite studies of all time (geek alert), researchers at the Ohio State University brought couples into the lab and had them engage in a marital conflict. But before they started the discussion, the researchers gave each member of the couple a small puncture wound on the arm! (Here's a shout-out to the many wonderful research volunteers out there who sign up for these and other studies to advance science, even when it involves personal discomfort.) The central research question was: Do certain behaviors (e.g., hostility) within couples predict slower wound healing? What is so elegant about this study is not only that they got couples to do it, but that wound healing is an excellent marker of our bodies' ability to fight off infection and our risk for other chronic health conditions, including cancer and heart disease.

The results were striking. Couples who showed a high level of hostility during the conflict (e.g., rolling eyes, criticizing the partner) healed at 60 percent of the rate of couples who were low in hostility. Mind you: all couples were instructed to discuss a "hot" topic in their relationship, so this is a perfect example to emphasize yet again that it is not the presence of conflict per se that is toxic for couples, but rather it's how you engage in conflict. Being nasty to your spouse or being treated nastily literally hurts the mind and body. And lack of sleep can make the health effects even worse. In a subsequent study, these same researchers found that couples who were struggling with sleep problems and who showed hostile behaviors in the conflict task showed particularly high levels of inflammatory markers associated with chronic disease. Talk about a toxic dance!

THE "LOVE HORMONE": OXYTOCIN

Oxytocin is a hormone produced in the brain and is most widely known for being released during childbirth or lactation. But both men and women produce oxytocin. Oxytocin is considered the "love hormone" because it is released during activities that are thought to promote pair bonding or affiliative behaviors, including sex or even while holding hands with a romantic partner. The release of oxytocin has also been shown to reduce the body's stress response, including lowering blood pressure levels and cortisol, and to promote pleasant feelings, including relaxation, so it likely plays an important role in facilitating sleep. However, there is strikingly little research available on the role of oxytocin and sleep, aside from a handful of studies in mice that were inconclusive. The burning question remains: Does naturally released oxytocin, stimulated by human contact and particularly through orgasm, promote relaxation and lead to better-quality and deeper sleep? Perhaps oxytocin is the underlying scientific explanation for the widely held though barely investigated belief that sex is good for sleep.

In an Australian study, 460 adults completed a survey including questions about their sex lives and sleep habits. About two-thirds of respondents said they slept much better after having an orgasm shortly before bed, which may be due to the release of oxytocin and other endorphins that accompany orgasms. Given that this data is based on self-report, it's hard to say whether oxytocin-release drove the self-reported benefits to sleep, or maybe the people who reported having an orgasm before bed were just happier and responded more positively to the survey. At this point, only a handful of studies have looked at how oxytocin influences sleep in humans, and their results are mixed. Clearly, there is a need to rigorously and systematically study the hormonal pathways linking sex with sleep, but such an undertaking, particularly in a laboratory setting, is challenging. (Although I could imagine several amorous partners trying to convince the other to participate in such a study: "Come on, honey. It's for science!")

Perhaps the strongest evidence in favor of sex as a sleep aid is that when couples engage in sex, it at least keeps them from doing the many other non–sleep promoting, and frankly non–relationship promoting, activities in bed like scrolling through Facebook, reading emails, or worrying about all the things they need to get done the next day.

Having a healthy sex life is also critical for a healthy relationship, although, just like the literal meaning of "sleeping together," which I'm discussing in this book, there is no one-size-fits-all recommendation for how much or when couples should be having sex. That is a couple-level decision. But if sex is being sacrificed for binge-watching Netflix or scrolling through Instagram posts, or if you're simply too tired all the time to even consider a romantic interlude, then it's probably time to take a step back and start prioritizing sleep to support your individual health and the health of your relationship.

COUPLES IN CONTEXT

It is important to recognize that how couples engage with each other, how they sleep, and how sleep and relationships interact are also influenced by other factors operating within each individual, such as personality characteristics or pre-existing mental or physical health problems, as well as by broader social factors, including couples' socioeconomic resources, their race and ethnicity, where they live, what type of work they do, the stressors they are exposed to, their access to health care, and so on. These broader contextual factors can serve as risk or protective factors that may intensify or mitigate the toxic dance between poor sleep and relationship quality.

Sleep, like virtually every other health outcome, is socially patterned, meaning that we see disproportionate rates of sleep problems based on race and ethnicity, with African Americans, Hispanics, and American Indians/Alaska Natives showing higher rates of sleep problems than their non-Hispanic white counterparts. We also see that individuals who are socioeconomically disadvantaged having higher rates of sleep problems than those of higher socioeconomic status.

Substantial research also shows that where people live plays a fundamental role in shaping their health and well-being, including their sleep health. People who live in unsafe or socioeconomically disadvantaged neighborhoods have higher rates of sleep problems as well as poorer physical health in general, including risk for diabetes and heart disease, in part because of reduced access to health-promoting resources like parks or safe places to walk. They also have greater exposure to stressors, like violence, crime, and, particularly for certain racial and ethnic minority populations, exposure to discrimination and racism. Feeling safe at night is critical to be able to fall into deep, restful sleep. The quality of one's closest relationship can play a big role in contributing to feelings of safety and security, but so too can the conditions and quality of one's neighborhood.

In turn, the toxic dance between relationship problems and sleep problems can be intensified in couples facing financial strain, as they may have less access to resources to cope with sleep or relationship issues. Solutions like sleeping in separate beds, keeping children in separate rooms, controlling the temperature in the bedroom, sleeping on a regular schedule, and more: they just don't match up with the reality of their lives.

Many of these broader social inequities are beyond the control of any individual couple, as they require systemic change, but that doesn't mean that better sleep and better relationships are reserved for those with all of life's advantages. If couples focus on addressing what they can control in their own relationships and sleep, they can make both better, and in doing so they may even find a powerful way to buffer against some of the negative consequences of these broader social influences.

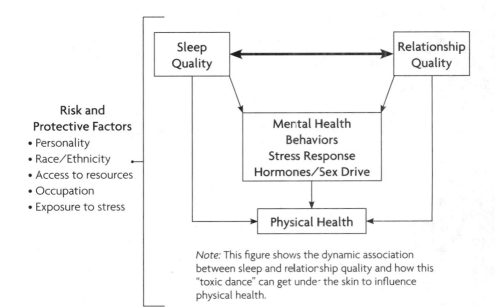

Note: This figure shows the dynamic association between sleep and relationship quality and how this "toxic dance" can get under the skin to influence physical health.

SHARED SLEEP ACTION PLAN:
Pillow Talk Ritual

In this chapter, we explored the interconnectedness between relationship quality, sleep quality, and various aspects of our health. If you take anything away from this chapter, it's that working to bolster your sleep or your relationship quality can bolster the other, and individually or collectively they can both bolster your health. However, neglecting either your sleep or your relationship can lead to a slippery slope toward poor health.

For this contribution to your Shared Sleep Action Plan, I want to try an exercise that many couples find valuable. As I discussed earlier, research shows that couples who are able to share their personal thoughts and feelings with their partner experience better sleep quality. That makes sense, as such open and honest sharing is a hallmark of a quality relationship. To help you build a habit around that behavior, I want to offer you a simple practice you can bring to your shared bed every night. (If you don't share beds, you can still come together before you go your separate ways for the night and have this moment together.)

The practice is called High, Low, Compliment, and it's simple. You and your partner lie down together and take turns sharing what you felt was the highest point in the day and the lowest point in the day, and then you give your partner a compliment. The highs or lows needn't necessarily be about your relationship, but they might be, and this is a time to discuss such feelings openly and honestly. This isn't about starting a fight. It's simply about sharing how you felt during the day. For the compliment, challenge yourself to find something different each day. Perhaps you noticed something your partner did particularly well. Or perhaps you just want to share something you enjoy about them. In relationships, especially long-term ones, we may say, "I love you," but we don't often say why. This is your opportunity to identify one of the many little reasons why.

High. Low. Compliment. Do this every night for a week. If you find after a few nights that having such discussions before bed leads either one of you to become upset or anxious or veering toward conflict, then that's probably a good sign to practice this exercise at a different time of day. Find the time that works best for both of you. At the end of the week, check in with each other to see how it feels. If you want, keep the practice for the long haul. It might just make you happier, healthier, and more rested.

chapter four

A VIRTUOUS CYCLE

ALYSSA AND CALVIN ARE DEAR FRIENDS OF MINE. AT THE WRITING of this, they have been married for over eighteen years and have three children ages eleven, fourteen, and sixteen. Over dinner one evening, we got to talking about how their sleep had evolved as their family evolved over time. (Isn't that what everyone talks about at dinner?) They told me that they had been sleeping on the same mattress for the entire duration of their marriage. When they casually revealed this fact to me, I couldn't withhold my surprise and dismay. "Eighteen years on the same mattress? What do you think, that these things have a lifetime guarantee?" I asked.

The general rule of thumb (at least according to the mattress industry, so take that with a grain of salt) is that mattresses should be replaced about every seven to ten years. Some beds might last longer than that, but eighteen years? Not likely. They were due for a replacement. Both Calvin and Alyssa are runners, so I explained to them, "Think of your mattress as the running shoes you're going to wear as you train for your next marathon. You want the best gear you can afford, to promote performance and reduce risk of injury. Same goes for your mattress."

Soon after, they took my advice and purchased a new mattress. "I honestly couldn't believe what a difference such a simple thing could make," said Calvin. "Now that I see the difference, I don't think I actually slept, like really slept, in the past ten years! Suddenly, I actually am having dreams and I wake up feeling refreshed." Before long, he and Alyssa also started to see some benefits in their relationship. "That bed that we had for so long, from the time we were newlyweds to when we were sleep-deprived parents of little ones, was about as far from a marital bed as you could imagine," Alyssa admitted. "It was definitely not sexy. It sounds silly, but something about investing in this new mattress, that was just for us, kind of marked this new stage in our marriage. Like okay, we got through the craziness of having young children in our home—and often in our bed—and now we are investing in us again." As they both started sleeping better, their moods improved, they felt less irritable, they "didn't sweat the small stuff with each other quite so much," and they were generally nicer to be around. And all that led to spending more time in bed together, more talking, more cuddling, more intimacy.

Replacing a mattress seems like a pretty simple fix, and frankly, for Alyssa and Calvin, it was, but for others, the causes of sleep problems may be more complicated or less under your control. But with all the things that can go wrong in your relationship when you skimp on sleep, there is an upshot to this feedback loop between the quality of your sleep and the quality of your relationship.

Taking even small steps to improve sleep can make a big difference in improving the quality of your relationship.

Because we live in a culture that continues to ascribe to the fatally flawed belief that sleep is an optional behavior or some sort of luxury to be pursued only when everything else is squared away, I feel that it is my professional obligation to tell anyone who will listen how important it is to prioritize sleep, not just for personal health, well-being, and productivity but also for relationship health. The problem with hammering home that important message is that it can also make people who are having trouble sleeping worried about what that might be doing to them. For that reason, when I begin work with my insomnia patients, while I acknowledge that there are serious consequences of not sleeping well, I also empha-size that *worrying* about those consequences does nothing to solve the problem. "Replace the worry with actionable steps," I encour-age them. I take the same approach here. By prioritizing sleep as a couple, really making it part of your shared value system, you and your partner can both realize the many benefits that come from a good night's sleep. These benefits will be reaped by both of you and will feed back into a virtuous cycle of healthy sleep leading to healthy relationships, and so on.

So what are these sleep-induced relationship benefits? Let's start with the superficial: When you sleep better, you look better. And looks matter. Physical attraction matters when trying to attract a mate. It also matters in long-term relationships.

Swedish researchers showed subjects photos of people who had been deprived of sleep and those who had sufficient sleep, and sub-jects rated the people in the sleep-deprived photos as less attractive and less healthy. Another study by University of Michigan research-ers found that patients with obstructive sleep apnea (OSA) were rated by both "lay observers" and medical professionals as being more youthful, alert, and attractive after receiving treatment for OSA. For many, the very idea of wearing "the Darth Vader mask" (the affectionate name commonly extolled for the front-line treatment for OSA—continuous positive airway pressure) is a major deterrent to adhering to this effective and health-promoting treatment. But these results demonstrate that letting this sleep problem go untreated can exact a real toll on your physical attraction. Beauty sleep is a real thing.

The relationship benefits of healthy sleep go well beyond skin-deep, affecting your health and your interpersonal skills. For example, studies have shown that sleep loss can contribute to expanding waistlines, with the strongest relationships observed among younger people. People who don't sleep enough or who have poor quality sleep tend to eat more (particularly carbohydrate and calorie-laden, high-fat foods, not carrot sticks) and have higher body mass indexes.

In Chapter 3, I described how sleep loss and sleep problems can send you galloping off with the Four Horsemen of the Apocalypse, to use the terminology from John Gottman's extensive relationship research (or in other words, the four tell-tale characteristics of relationships on a fast track to rupture). Of course, there are many relationship theories and experts out there, but I find Gottman's work especially useful in this context because it provides a framework for considering the flip side: how healthy sleep can facilitate the positive relationship behaviors that are the antidote to toxic relationship behaviors.

In short, according to Gottman and his team's work on the factors that predict long-term, healthy relationships versus those that predict relationship demise, the antidotes to criticism, contempt, defensiveness, and stonewalling are, respectively, gentle start-up, build a culture of appreciation, take responsibility, and physiological self-soothing. Each of these antidotes can be thought of as skills. Some people may be naturally better at some of them than others, but regardless of where you begin, just about all of us can learn these skills, and getting the sleep you need can support the acquisition of such skills. Even more importantly, getting the sleep you need can promote your ability to implement them when needed most (e.g., in the midst of a heated conversation about your mother-in-law).

ANTIDOTE TO CRITICISM: START YOUR ENGINES—SLOWLY

One of the joys and challenges of being with another person for any extended period of time is that you really get to know their strengths and their weaknesses. Not to put too fine a point on it, but the more you know someone, the easier it can be to find their faults as well, which can lead to toxic relationship behavior number 1: criticism. When you skimp on sleep, being critical of the person you love comes far too easily, because you're more prone to negative moods, are more irritable, and have trouble seeing the other person's perspective. It bears repeating: having conflict with a partner is not a sign of an unhealthy relationship; it's how you engage in conflict that matters. In fact, the antidote to criticism is not avoidance of difficult topics or denial of your partner's real or perceived faults, but rather a softer, gentler approach to engaging in those tough and potentially hurtful topics.

The slow or "gentle start-up" technique turns blame or criticism of the other person into a reflection of your feelings, a skill that requires emotion regulation, good communication skills, and the ability to inhibit knee-jerk reactions—all supported by healthy sleep. For example, instead of saying, "You never put your family's needs first. It's all about you and your work," the gentle start-up might sound something like this: "I understand that your work is really stressful, but I need you, and our family needs you. I'd like it if you could be more involved with us." The latter, relationship-enhancing example uses "I" statements and focuses on your feelings and expresses what you want, but in a positive way. Easier said than done, right? But as I said, it's a skill to be practiced and one that you will be much more able to access if you are well-rested, since sleep supports healthy communication skills and good judgment, including knowing when to bring up a touchy topic or when to table it for another time.

Getting the sleep we need also supports our ability to use cognitive strategies, such as reappraisal—the ability to think about an upsetting situation or events from a more helpful or relationship-promoting way, including a slow start-up to difficult conversations. In one study participants reported on a number of dimensions of their sleep, including quality and duration over the past week, and were then asked to watch a series of sad films in the laboratory. After the films they were asked to "think about the situation you see in a more positive light," a technique used in research to elicit cognitive reappraisal. For example, after watching a film about a family dog dying, a cognitive reappraisal might involve thinking, *Well, that dog lived a happy life and was loved by his family*. This approach simply offers a new perspective on an otherwise very sad situation. It's not about being pollyannaish about the situation, but rather thinking about the situation in a way that brings more balance and potentially reduces the negative emotion at hand, whether sadness, anger, or fear. In this study, the researchers found that higher sleep quality was associated with higher levels of cognitive reappraisal.

This is a helpful skill in the context of relationships: reacting to your partner in the height of negative emotion rarely helps you achieve the goal of effective communication. Cognitive reappraisal is also an important strategy for dampening the intensity of negative emotions and likelihood of unleashing criticisms on your partner, which can lead to escalation of relationship conflict. For example, it's one thing if you see dirty dishes in the sink and appraise the situation as "yet another example of my husband not listening to my pleas or caring about my feelings" versus "I feel frustrated that he didn't clean up the dishes the way I asked, but maybe I need to find more effective ways of getting what I want."

ANTIDOTE FOR CONTEMPT: LITTLE ACTS OF LOVE

Contempt, which may include sarcasm, cynicism, name-calling, or hostile humor is the biggest predictor of divorce, according to Gottman's work, so definitely one to avoid. It's also important to strengthen the antidote of "building a culture of appreciation and respect." This sounds like a good idea, but what does it actually mean, and how does it relate to sleep?

As much as long-term relationships may be punctuated by major, shared life events and milestones, like getting married, having children, and buying your first house or apartment together, the foundation of a relationship is built on the small, everyday actions and interactions that you share with your partner. Building a culture of appreciation and respect is all about regularly expressing appreciation, gratitude, affection, and respect for the other person. Little acts of kindness or love can create a reserve account of positivity for both of you, and they can also serve as a buffer to reduce the likelihood of contempt bubbling up. These relational building blocks also serve as a powerful reminder of the core tenet of any healthy relationship: that even though things may get tough and you may get angry with each other, you hold the other person's feelings in the palm of your hand, as they do yours. Expressions of contempt, on the other hand, are the ultimate violation of that tenet.

Research has shown that couples who slept better over a period of two weeks were more thankful for each others' thoughtful behaviors and less selfish. On the other hand, people reported feeling less appreciated if either they *or* their partner slept poorly. This is yet another reminder of the importance of prioritizing sleep *as a couple*. If either one of you is not sleeping well, it could send you both into a tailspin of feeling underappreciated and uncared for.

Lead author of the study, Dr. Amie Gordon, emphasizes the importance of these findings and notes that "showing our partners we care and are grateful for the things they do for us is vital in any healthy relationship."

As chaotic as many of our lives are, the bedroom is a great location to regularly and routinely practice such small acts that contribute to a culture of appreciation and respect. Simply lying quietly with each other before bed, holding hands, cuddling, having sex, or making sure that the first thing you say to each other when you wake up is "Good morning" and looking at each other when doing so can go a long way to reminding both of you that you are in this together.

For couples who choose to sleep apart, it's still possible and absolutely essential to take advantage of these moments. For example, some couples will choose to share their bedtime ritual together in one room, then go their separate ways when it's time to sleep. Depending on schedules, other couples may choose to have a delicious reunion in the morning, to reconnect and punctuate the start of the day with kind words or a cuddle with the person they love.

Regardless of the sleeping arrangement, the key is to practice being present and mindful in these moments of peace and togetherness. There is no more powerful way to show the person you love that you are there for them and that you care than to simply be present during these rare, quiet moments. These acts of affection and kindness can also support you both getting healthy sleep by serving as a powerful buffer to the usual stresses of the day and a reminder that you have someone in your corner. Sleep, in turn, can also facilitate greater likelihood of practicing relationship-promoting behaviors by improving your mood, improving empathy, and improving your perspective-taking ability.

At a broader level, when you are well-slept, you are more likely to experience positive moods, you are funnier, are more fun to be around, and have more energy, which can mean you're more likely to engage in shared pleasurable activities together—a crucial factor in maintaining and sustaining long-term and happy relationships. Laughter, for example, can be a powerful aphrodisiac. Dr. Jeffrey Hall, a professor of communication studies at Kansas University, found that when a man and a woman who are strangers meet, the more times the man tries to be funny and the more the woman laughs at those efforts, the more likely it is for the woman to be interested in pursuing a relationship. But an even better predictor of romantic connection is if the two are spotted laughing together. In fact, humor is cited as one of the most valued traits in a romantic partner. Humor done well takes a great deal of cognitive precision, timing, and focus—skills that suffer dramatically when poorly slept. A study from Walter Reed Army Institute of Medical Research found that when subjects were sleep-deprived, they laughed less when viewing silly cartoons. (How sad.)

Whether or not you or your partner is a natural comedian, make time for shared experiences together that remind both of you that you chose each other. Life can be demanding, sometimes even grueling, but when you make time to share enjoyable experiences with your partner, you are reaffirming your choice that this is the person you choose to be with, so make time for the fun parts.

If I haven't convinced you already that prioritizing your sleep is one of the best investments you can make in your relationship, based on the demonstrated positive effects of sleep on healthy communication skills, empathy, and humor, not to mention your mental and physical health (including your brain health), how about more and better sex? According to a study of more than 170 women, published in the *Journal of Sexual Medicine*, for every extra hour of sleep (over a two-week period), women were 14 percent more likely to engage in sexual activity with a partner.

ANTIDOTE TO DEFENSIVENESS: OWNING YOUR SCREW-UPS

None of us are perfect. We all make mistakes, big and small, in our relationships. Most people value their relationships, so even minor ways that we disappoint our partners can feel pretty bad, leading to shame and guilt. The question is, How do you respond when you screw up? Do you get defensive (Horseman number 3), or do you own up to your mistake and take responsibility, which is the antidote to defensiveness?

Taking responsibility is one of those adult sorts of behaviors that requires you to have your wits about you, including the ability to see both sides of the situation and stand in your partner's shoes. Research has shown that getting adequate duration and quality sleep supports these very adult relationships.

One of the first tenets of relationship therapy is "don't expect your partner to be a mind reader," and that is great advice. Your partner can't always know exactly what you are feeling, so rather than wishing they knew you were feeling down about your day, it's always a helpful strategy just to tell them! That said, one of the powerful ways of connecting with another human being is feeling that they understand what it's like to be in your shoes and empathize with how you are feeling. Research has shown that while healthy sleep can't turn you into a mind reader, it can make you more aware of your partner's feelings and more able to regulate your own feelings. This can be a vastly important attribute in a relationship. When you can read your partner's experiences and emotions and effectively manage your own emotions, you can respond in a nondefensive manner and take responsibility where it is warranted. "I'm feeling really hurt, but I can tell that what I said really hurt you. I don't want to hurt you. I'm sorry for that." It can also help you avoid the tyranny of being in the right, an affliction many of us have, which rarely if ever benefits the relationship.

The thing about defensiveness is that it is literally that: a defense reaction. When we feel threatened or attacked, it is natural to initially feel defensive and to do anything we can to avoid the unpleasant experience of feeling blamed. Because sleep loss is experienced as a threat to the system and can cause elevations in physiological stress responses, being poorly slept can lead to heightened feelings of vigilance and greater perceived threat in our environments, which can set us up for greater likelihood of responding in a defensive manner.

ANTIDOTE TO STONEWALLING: CALM THE F*CK DOWN

When stress gets so intense that the person feels overwhelmed or flooded with emotion, they tend to check out and withdraw to protect themselves. This would be the Horseman known as stonewalling. It goes back to the fight-or-flight response; only this time it's your partner who is the perceived threat, not a saber-toothed tiger. The flooding of emotions and physiological reactivity stemming from relationship conflict can lead to an especially toxic relationship dynamic known as demand-withdraw. In this dynamic, one partner is perceived as the attacker, while the other becomes increasingly overwhelmed by negative emotions and their own stress response. When under such attack, and feeling emotionally overwhelmed and stressed out, a person will often shut down and completely disengage as a means of protecting themselves.

Getting good sleep helps us smooth out our emotional edges, making us less reactive and less likely to escalate conflicts with our partner. A team of scientists from the University of California, Berkeley, have shown that a good night of sleep may function as a bit of overnight therapy, helping you to selectively forget some of the negative experiences that happen during the day. If not addressed, these negative memories cumulatively can increase your risk for mood disorders, like depression or anxiety, and we know that mental health problems are a primary source of relationship stress and relationship rupture. This is yet another reason to prioritize your sleep.

In Gottman's early work, he and his colleagues tested out their hypothesis about the causal relationship between emotional and physiological flooding and stonewalling in a clever way. First, couples were asked to engage in an argument, as with many other laboratory experiments of couples' interactions. Then, about fifteen minutes into the argument, the experimenter interrupted and told the couple that she (the experimenter) had to leave the room to fix some of the equipment. This interruption was, in fact, the key manipulation of the experiment. The equipment was fine, but during the interruption the couple was asked to stop talking and just read magazines for a half hour, providing them with a half-hour break or cool-down period from each other. Once the experimenter returned to the room, and the couple was asked to reengage, their heart rates (which were being measured throughout the experiment) were significantly lower, and their interaction was more productive and positive. Such a simple manipulation provided an opportunity for the couple to physiologically self-regulate or self-soothe and ultimately engage in a healthier form of conflict, even though the couple wasn't aware that an intervention had occurred.

Sleep deprivation and sleep problems, including insomnia, only serve to make a bad situation worse, as insufficient or otherwise disturbed sleep is known to disrupt both emotional and physiological self-regulation. Healthy sleep, on the other hand, is one of nature's best salves for the biting sting of raw emotions and nerves. Getting the sleep you need provides the reserves and the resources to show yourself and your partner the compassion you so desperately need when you are under stress, including the stress of conflict. When you can access such compassion, you can tap into your own self-regulatory skills to know when to say "when," including calling a temporary break to the conversation (just as the experimenters in Gottman's work did), to catch your breath, gather your wits, and down-regulate some of that stress response.

But what happens when tempers flare right before bedtime? We've all heard the old adage "Don't go to bed angry," but what's a couple to do? Should they stay up and try to douse the flames of conflict, or let the emotions simmer and table the conflict for another time? In 2011, researchers from the University of Utah found that anger before bedtime did not lead to sleep disruption among couples; however, couple conflict before bedtime did disrupt sleep. In other words, technically the correct adage is not "don't go to bed angry," but rather, "don't fight before bed." It's not anger that's the problem; it's the conflict anger creates. This is good news for couples because the reality is that many problems couples face cannot be tidily resolved in time for bed. Choose your battles and the timing of those battles. A fight before bedtime is unlikely to be resolved and may rob you both of sleep. If conflict is escalating and either one of you is feeling flooded with emotions, it could be beneficial to tell your partner, "I care about this too much to continue fighting when we are both exhausted and don't have our wits about us. Let's table this for tonight and return to it tomorrow, when we both are going to be better at working through things." This is also the time to practice self-care, like meditating or taking a walk so you can de-escalate your own physiological arousal and then go to sleep. No good will come out of the continued argument when you are both tired.

SHARED SLEEP ACTION PLAN:
Promoting a Virtuous Sleep and Relationship Cycle

There are many ways to put that virtuous cycle in motion, which I discuss throughout this book, but here I want to focus on some physical changes you can make to your shared sleep environment to send the message that sleep is a priority for both of you. Even if you don't sleep together, you should determine as a couple that a particular place is your shared haven, where you can share the time together before falling asleep, first thing in the morning, or perhaps just some afternoon delights if you are so able and inclined. Too often our bedrooms are becoming cluttered extensions of our already cluttered and chaotic lives, replete with phones and tablets on our nightstand, laundry on the floor, and maybe even children's toys scattered about. It's time to reclaim your space and make your bedroom a haven. Here's how.

1. **Invest in a good mattress.** Remember that we spend roughly one-third of our lives asleep, so it is worth putting a premium on the comfort of your sleeping arrangement. Spend what you can afford within your budget, but don't skimp out on this luxury, as you are going to be spending a lot of time on it. The key is comfort for you and your partner, so to the extent possible, try out your mattress first. Many mattress companies extend generous return policies so that you have the opportunity to test one out, and don't have to feel stuck if you change your mind. Personally, I have been a fan of the hotel brand beds, because I found that the best way for me to try out the product was based on my prior experiences sleeping exceptionally well in certain hotel beds. As I told Alyssa and Calvin, mattresses have a shelf-life and need to be replaced every seven to ten years.

2. **Make yourself a tidy and inviting nest.** I am a scientist, not an interior designer, so while I am no expert in the trendiest or most stylish room decor, I can tell you that there are some science-backed, basic dos and don'ts when it comes to turning your bedroom into a haven for sleep. In terms of colors, neutrals, silvers, and greys have been shown to be relaxing and

can even lower your blood pressure and heart rate. Splashes of color, particularly if they make you happy or feel warm and inviting are also acceptable, but just don't make it too bright, as that can be alerting. Beyond the color palette, what's even more important is what you keep in your room and what you keep out. You want your haven to be free from clutter and the distractions of the day—that includes dirty laundry scattered on the floor or your phone by your bedside. All that detritus sends the wrong signal to the brain and can increase anxiety. The bedroom should be for sleep and sex—keep it simple and inviting. And when you wake up in the morning, set yourself up for sleep that subsequent night by making your bed first thing. Each night that you return to bed should be an invitation to your warm, inviting, and tidy haven.

3. **Keep your relationship hot, but the bedroom cool.** As we sleep, our body temperatures naturally decline. In fact, a dip in core body temperature is a key signal to our brains that it's time to fall asleep. Generally speaking, the recommendation is to keep your bedroom between about 65 to 68 degrees, which is much colder than many of us would naturally feel comfortable in during the daytime. The goal is not to have you shivering all night. Make sure you have enough blankets that can come on or off as needed to regulate your temperature throughout the night. Setting your thermostat a bit cooler than normal can gently nudge your body temperature to dip, which facilitates your ability to fall into deep, restful sleep. There is even some truth to the old adage about a warm bath being good for sleep for this very reason. While you're in the bath, your temperature rises, but it falls precipitously when you get out. Try a bath about ninety minutes before bedtime.

Better yet—do it with your partner, and make it a part of your shared bedtime ritual. It's a great way to relax and unwind with each other and reduce your body temperature (provided that things don't get too steamy).

4. **It's better in the dark.** While some may argue whether sex is better in the light of day or in total darkness, there is no question that sleep is better when the lights are down. Sometimes this is more than simply turning off the light switch. Make sure if light creeps in through the window that you use blinds or drapes or even hang a dark sheet over the window if necessary. If some light cannot be avoided, or if you and your partner are on different schedules, with one coming to bed later, consider wearing an eye mask. And it goes without saying but must be repeated that if the light is coming from a phone or other electronic device in the hands of your partner or yourself, get that sleep stealer out of the bedroom. Light in general, but particularly the blue light that comes from electronic devices, directly suppresses the hormone melatonin, which signals the brain that it is time for sleep. And before you go excusing your device because you have a blue-light filter, let me just say that it is also the stimulating content that we consume from our devices, not just the light that can keep us up at night. Set the mood (for sleep and maybe even a little romance) by turning the lights down in the evening, a couple hours before bedtime, as dim lights can also stimulate the release of melatonin and set you up for sleep success that night.

5. **Punctuate the start and end of the day with small but sweet gestures.** Bringing your partner coffee in the morning or giving your partner a backrub as they wake up or go to

sleep, even when you are tired and cranky and irritable, can go a long way toward building goodwill and compassion in your relationship. It's like putting money in your relationship bank account. You may not be a great conversationalist, and you may be snappy, but these small gestures of kindness can smooth out those edges. It may surprise you how these small acts can make you and your partner feel better and can start or end the day a little brighter.

chapter five

HIS, HERS, AND OUR SLEEP

ALEX AND SYLVIA ARE BOTH IN THEIR SIXTIES, HAPPILY MARRIED, and enjoying their lives as empty nesters, since their three grown children have successfully launched their own independent lives. After thirty-five years of marriage, their sleep routine is pretty stable. It goes something like this: They get into bed around ten p.m., they watch the nightly news, and by eleven p.m. it's lights out. That's when the drama really unfolds. Alex falls asleep. The snoring begins. And not just any snoring. Loud, halting, rattling, almost inhuman snoring. Sylvia lies there, wide awake and in agony. Her usual sweet and loving self devolves into bitterness, frustration, and, ultimately, downright fury. When his snorts and excruciatingly loud exhales finally get the best of her, she lashes out with a fierce jab to his ribs. He awakens, momentarily, sleepily gives a barely intelligible, "What did I do?" before falling back to sleep. His snoring resumes, and her insomnia also resumes.

This story is true. Sylvia and Alex are real. But I could have just as easily substituted their names with Jesse and Joseph, Alison and Michael, Lexi and William, or a multitude of other couples I've worked with or researched. This story of an insomniac wife struggling to sleep alongside a loudly snoring husband—it's *the* common story when it comes to couples and poor sleep. Now before anyone claims I am being sexist by blaming this on the male partner, I readily admit that women, too, can be the culprit in this nightly drama. But statistically speaking, men are about twice as likely to be snorers or at least loud snorers as compared to women (although the field levels off somewhat as women go through menopause). Women, on the other hand, are more likely to suffer from insomnia. It's easy to assume that a partner's snoring causes the insomnia, but it's also possible that the snoring simply exacerbates the insomnia and provides a convenient target of blame for the individual with insomnia to direct her rage. One partner can't sleep. The other partner is snoring loudly. The sleepless partner builds contempt for that snore and for the snorer. That contempt makes it even harder to sleep, and if it goes on for long enough, it can potentially harm the relationship. And of course, this can play out in same-sex couples as well, since both men and women can be snorers or have insomnia. Vicious cycle.

I would (and did) advise Sylvia to talk to her husband about his snoring, because it could be a sign of a serious health problem. He could be suffering from obstructive sleep apnea (about 50 percent of snorers have it), which is a potentially dangerous condition. But if curing her insomnia was as simple as turning off the snore, I'd have told her to purchase some really good ear plugs and move on. It's often not that simple. Addressing problems like the inability to fall asleep or stay asleep or getting quality, restful sleep often requires more than that. And if you're looking to improve sleep for you and your partner, it first requires looking inward. That's because how you sleep as a couple is heavily influenced by how you each sleep as individuals. And how we all sleep as individuals is often greatly influenced by how we live our lives as well as by our biology.

There are some habits and behaviors that help promote sleep. There are some habits and behaviors that get in the way of sleep. If you and your partner are looking to improve your shared sleep, you might start by looking at how well, or not well, your individual habits and behaviors are working for you. If your lifestyle or certain behaviors are keeping you from sleeping as well as you'd like, it's possible the resulting tossing and turning, snoring, or other disturbances you're creating aren't helping your partner's sleep much either.

Sleep researchers refer to these habits and behaviors as sleep hygiene. There's evidence to suggest that practicing good sleep hygiene can go a long way to helping you improve your sleep — although it is rarely sufficient to treat full-blown insomnia. The following table explores those factors that most heavily influence your ability to get to sleep and stay asleep. As you look at them, reflect on your own patterns and practices. Are some of your habits actually creating a problem for you and potentially for your partner?

FACTORS THAT INFLUENCE SLEEP
(OR CONTRIBUTE TO A LACK OF IT)

Caffeine	It seems obvious to say it, but caffeine gets in the way of sleep. Caffeine can stay in your system for several hours. My recommendation is to avoid caffeinated beverages or foods anytime after two or three in the afternoon. Caffeine is, of course, found in coffee. It's also in teas, colas, energy drinks, chocolate, and even some pain relievers. We all process caffeine somewhat differently, so experimenting a bit with when and how much caffeine you consume in any given day as well as tracking your sleep is a great way to figure out what's working and not working for you. And here's a tip: many of us like a nighttime dessert (I consider it essential), but beware of chocolate. For many, consuming too much or too rich chocolate at night can lead to a sleepless night.
Nicotine	Nicotine is found in cigarettes and e-cigarettes and is also a stimulant, so it can make it hard to fall asleep or cause your sleep to be less restful. Smoking doesn't help sleep in any way, and it's disastrous for your health, so now you have yet another reason to quit.
Alcohol	It is true that alcohol in high enough quantities can help you fall asleep. However, as your body processes the sugars in the alcohol throughout the night, it can deliver a burst of energy that wakes you up, and then you can struggle to get back to sleep.
Food	Having a big meal late at night can cause problems for sleep. A lighter meal four hours or more before bedtime is better for sleep. The key here is you don't want your belly to be too full or too empty before bed, so that's why a light, healthful snack, like a piece of fruit, a glass of milk, or a handful of almonds is the way to go, when it comes to a snack before bedtime.

Mobile Devices	Mobile devices are ruining our sleep (among other things). Not only is it easy to lose track of time while checking out Instagram, but the light these devices emit disrupts sleep by suppressing the hormone melatonin, which signals the brain that it's time to sleep. Just having your phone nearby while you sleep can be disruptive because it is such a potent reminder of our waking lives and all the stress and demands that come with that. My best advice is to keep your phone and other screens out of your bedroom. And if you have children or teenagers in the home, it's especially important that you model good behaviors, including keeping technology out of the bedroom, because your kids are watching. Studies have shown that parents who keep their phones in their bedroom are more likely to have kids who have phones in their bedroom. So model this healthy behavior for the whole family.
Temperature	We sleep better in a cool space, and that's partly because a drop in body temperature is one of the key changes that happens as we fall asleep. Keeping the room cool and even nudging your body along toward this drop in body temperature (e.g., by taking a warm bath before bed) can facilitate your ability to fall asleep and stay asleep. The ideal temperature is somewhere around 65 to 68 degrees, give or take a few degrees. That's not always attainable, so do what you can to make your bedroom as cool as possible to help bring on sleep. You also don't want to be shivering throughout the night, so it's better to keep the room temperature cool but layer up with blankets, which you can throw off as needed. This is especially important for women as they transition through menopause and experience the joys of hot flashes. And for couples who have different temperature preferences, this is also where having separate covers for each partner is key.
Sense of Security and Comfort	It's hard to sleep if you feel at risk in your bed. The research shows that people who live in areas with more crime have poorer sleep We don't always get to pick where we live. Simple things like having good locks on your doors and windows can go a long way to giving you the security you need to sleep well. Also, investing in a high-quality mattress and bedding, and reducing clutter in your bedroom, can help create a comfortable and relaxing environment to promote healthy sleep. Of course, feeling safe and secure in your relationship can also facilitate your ability to sleep.

continues

Exercise	If you ask me, exercise is a panacea for just about anything that ails you, and that includes sleep. Even small bouts of daily exercise can go a long way to improving your sleep. Although the effects of nighttime exercise vary from individual to individual, for most people it's generally wise to avoid too strenuous or socially stimulating (e.g., at a gym) workouts too close to bedtime. Experiment with the timing of exercise that works best for you, but commit to engaging in some physical activity on a daily basis. It's good for your sleep and good for your mind and body.
Darkness at Night/ Lots of Light During the Day	You want your room as dark as possible to help bring on sleep. Do what you can to eliminate all light. That includes light from windows and from your devices. It all serves to block sleep. Even dimming the lights in your house in the evening hours before bedtime can make it easier to fall asleep at night, because dim lights facilitate the release of melatonin. During the daytime, however, particularly first thing in the morning, get as much light as possible. Natural light is preferred, so open the curtains, and get outside as much as possible. Light exposure during the daytime signals the brain that it's time to be alert and awake and can boost your energy and mood, setting you up for a good night of sleep when bedtime arrives. If you work nights or irregular shifts, and must sleep during daylight, it is especially important to block out as much light as possible, to help "trick" your brain that it is actually time for sleep.
Routine	Potentially one of the most important factors that influences your sleep is when you sleep. Ideally you'd go to bed *and* wake up at the same time every day—even on the weekends. And if you have to choose one over the other, a consistent wake time is the most important. Wake-up time is a critically important cue for setting our internal biological clock. Wake-up time also influences when we get exposed to light, and light is a powerful signal to the brain that it's time to start the day. So setting a consistent wake-up time is a good first step to setting you up for sleep success that night.

It's important to evaluate your personal behaviors that affect your sleep because of course, to some extent, we are all unique snowflakes when it comes to how we sleep and what best supports our sleep quality. Developing an understanding of your personal sleep profile, including your vulnerabilities for certain types of sleep problems, the consequences of sleep loss, what helps you unwind and what keeps you up at night, when you sleep best, and your specific habits and behaviors around sleep, is important work to do to improve your sleep.

It's also helpful to recognize that one of the biggest factors that influences our sleep in general is our biologically based sex as well as our socioculturally influenced gender. Some of the challenges that heterosexual couples face when sharing a bed stem from these sex- or gender-based differences in sleep. Even how men and women respond to sleep loss differs. For example, in a laboratory study of sleep deprivation, a team of Italian researchers found that after a night of sleep deprivation, men made riskier decisions in a laboratory gambling task, whereas women did the opposite—they made less risky decisions, relative to their well-slept state. Can you imagine how this might make it hard to see eye to eye with your partner if your behaviors following skimping on sleep go in completely opposite directions?

THE GENDER GAP IN SLEEP: THE PARADOX OF SLEEP QUANTITY VERSUS QUALITY

Now that we understand some of the individual-level behaviors that can help or hinder sleep regardless of sex and gender, let's shift to looking at how men and women experience sleep differently and how this contributes to specific sleep challenges faced by heterosexual couples. Taking time to consider how your and your partner's sleep is shaped by your sex and gender is a critical step in finding ways to overcome challenges in the bedroom. Doing so can help you both develop some compassion and understanding for each other, and it can even present opportunities for compromise and creative problem solving. So let's explore how men and women tend to differ when it comes to sleep.

First, men are two to three times more likely to have the clinical disorder known as obstructive sleep apnea (OSA). Snoring, when it is a symptom of OSA, is much more than just a nuisance; it can be a risk factor for major chronic health conditions, like heart disease and stroke.

There are a number of reasons why men are at greater risk for OSA compared to women. Anatomically, men tend to have narrower air passages as compared to women, as well as thicker necks. In fact, college and professional football players are a high-risk group for OSA, relative to other athletes. Just look at the size of their necks as one potential risk factor. When airways are narrow and necks are thick, this makes it harder for air to flow during normal inhalations and exhalations throughout the night, and when the air has to pass through a narrow opening and there is a lot of flesh around the neck, this can result in more intense vibrations in the tissue, resulting in even louder snoring.

Lifestyle factors, including alcohol use and smoking, also play a role in the gender gap in snoring. Men are more likely to use alcohol and to be heavy alcohol users as compared to women. Alcohol can cause the muscles in the neck to relax, causing a narrowing of the airways and greater vibrations in the neck.

Smoking, too, is statistically more common in men. Not only is the nicotine in tobacco products a stimulant, but smoking can cause inflammation in the airways, contributing to increased risk of snoring. As if we needed yet another reason never to smoke or to quit.

How men and women carry excess body weight also contributes to men's greater risk of snoring. In the US, as a society as a whole, we are losing the battle of the bulge, with about two-thirds of adults being overweight or obese, based on body mass index classifications. That said, men are more likely than women to carry their extra pounds in their upper body, including their chests and necks, which can increase the risk for loud snoring at night.

But the gender gap in sleep goes beyond snoring alone. While men run the greater risk of sleeping *loudly*, women are at greater risk of sleeping *poorly*. As I mentioned before, women are twice as likely to have clinical insomnia, which is characterized by difficulty falling or staying asleep, or poor-quality or nonrestorative sleep, despite adequate opportunity for sleep. In fact, it's one of nature's cruel jokes—at least for heterosexual couples. Pair a woman, the sex more prone to insomnia and therefore more susceptible to disrupted sleep, with a man, who is statistically more likely to snore, and the result is often that neither partner is sleeping well, and at least one partner (often the woman) is increasingly resentful.

Women are also at greater risk for restless legs syndrome (RLS), another sleep disorder that can make sleep more of a nightly battle than a peaceful respite. When I assess for RLS symptoms in new patients, many look at me kind of funny, because I ask, "Do you have creepy-crawly feelings or tingly sensations in your legs as you fall asleep or during sleep?" But those who have the symptoms know exactly what I am talking about. These creepy-crawly sensations can make it difficult to have a restful night of sleep: they cause a lot of discomfort, and the only relief comes from moving one's legs. Such movements can also have negative impacts on the bed partner's sleep. It's hard to get your rest when your partner's legs keep twitching.

Why women are more prone to these specific types of disorders than men is likely a combination of hormonal, physiological, and sociocultural factors. For example, women's risk of insomnia complaints often goes hand-in-hand with fluctuations in sex hormone production, such as during puberty, the menstrual cycle, pregnancy, postpartum, and the menopausal transition; however, the exact role of sex hormones in influencing women's risk is still not entirely clear.

Throughout my clinical career, I would estimate that at least half of my clients are women in their late forties to fifties, which is perhaps no surprise given substantial research showing a significant uptick in sleep problems among women approaching or going through menopausal transition. For example, studies have shown that sleep complaints are one of the most common symptoms reported by women as they go through menopausal transition, with 33 to 51 percent reporting such complaints. For many of my patients who are in the early stages of menopause, called perimenopause, when they still may be having periods but the periods become less regular, it is often a huge source of validation for them to learn that many studies have shown that perimenopause is often when sleep problems are at their worst—even relative to full-blown menopause. This can come as somewhat of a relief because many women fear that "if it's this bad now, then how bad can it possibly get when I actually start having hot flashes and the other joys of full-blown menopause?" Of course, I make no guarantees, and unfortunately, for some women the problems do persist and sometimes worsen, particularly when hot flashes are severe. Somewhat shockingly, given that the hormonal changes associated with puberty, pregnancy, and menopause affect 50 percent of the population, there is still a great deal of uncertainty about whether hormones or other factors are the driving force behind the spikes in sleep disturbances.

Making matters even more complicated is the fact that in studies in which sleep is measured objectively, we don't see the same steep declines in sleep quality throughout the menopausal transition that are reflected in women's reports. This discrepancy between women's reports of sleep complaints during menopause and the lack of objective sleep data to demonstrate an uptick in sleep problems is a paradox we see in general between men's and women's sleep. Despite having double the rates of insomnia as compared to men, when sleep is measured objectively, using polysomnography (which measures brain and muscle activity during sleep), women actually sleep longer and more deeply as compared to men. This paradox has sometimes been interpreted to mean that women just complain more than men, but new science is emerging that suggests that how we measure sleep—even with the current, "gold standard" sleep measurement, polysomnography, we might be missing something that is going on in women's brains during sleep.

When a more nuanced measurement of sleep is used, which measures the different types of brain activity that happen during each stage of sleep, called quantitative electro-encephalographic (QEEG) activity, the data suggests that even when women are asleep, parts of their brain are still actively processing information. This coheres perfectly with virtually every woman I've ever spoken to with insomnia who says, "Sometimes I feel like even if I'm asleep, my brain is still awake. It's as if there's a light that's still flickering in my brain, so it doesn't feel like I'm really asleep." Here's where I'm going to shift gears a bit and start referring to gender rather than sex differences, because this is where our differences are largely defined by the social roles associated with men and women, perhaps more so than our biological sex differences.

I saw an advertisement the other day that read, "Sleep like you did before you had children." Boy, did that get my attention. For many women, sleeping the way you did before you had children is like finding the Holy Grail. I can't tell you how many patients and friends have implored me, "Will I ever sleep the way I did before having kids?" With my own kids, I remember thinking once they were both solidly out of the middle-of-the-night-awakening-and-needing-mommy-or-daddy, *How unfair is this? Why am I still waking up at the drop of a hat, when my husband can seemingly sleep through everything?*

Our current situation is a perfect example. We recently got a new puppy, in part because my older dog is really anxious and I thought he could use a therapy dog to help him feel more comfortable socially. And in part, because, frankly, I miss having babies in the house (at least during the daytime). At night, it's been a whole different story, harkening back to those early days when my children were just infants. When the pup, Gus, makes the slightest whimper, I am awake in an instant. My husband sleeps. I will myself (sometimes successfully, sometimes not) to not feel resentful because I suspect that this might be, to some extent, an evolutionarily based difference in the sexes, as well as a socioculturally based difference in gender role expectations.

Recently, I had the opportunity to speak to Dr. Sarah Burgard, a sociologist and professor at the University of Michigan, about her work on gender differences in sleep. Her research explores how men and women differentially spend and prioritize their time, and how personal and cultural expectations about time use for men and women contribute to disparities we see in workforce participation as well as mental and physical well-being. From that vantage point, she became interested in sleep for several reasons. "First of all," she explained, "proportionally, sleep takes up a lot of our time, and as a sociologist, I am interested in how men and women use their time and how it relates to social roles. Secondly, even though sleep is a fundamental health behavior and a corner-stone of healthy minds and bodies, we tend to think of sleep as being a discretionary behavior. So how one prioritizes or doesn't prioritize sleep could absolutely fall along gendered lines." For example, women, especially if they are married and have children, spend more time doing unpaid work (much of which is household responsibilities) and less time in leisure activity, as compared to men. Therefore, sleep might be sacrificed in lieu of the other de-mands of unpaid work that disproportionately fall upon women. She went on to further explain how, when she and her colleagues first embarked on their study that examined over fifty thousand Americans, she fully expected that their work would be the first to debunk the prior research showing that women actually sleep more than men. She was convinced that their large, representative sample and use of rigorous time-use methods, which essentially involves having participants meticulously document all of their daily and nightly activities, including sleep, diary-style, over a twenty-four-hour period, would produce results that more accurately reflect the sleep experience of men and women in the real world. To her surprise, however, their results actually confirmed prior findings. Women, in their study, slept on average twenty-three minutes more than men. Once the researchers took into account the time men and women spent in paid or unpaid work, the gender difference favoring women's sleep duration persisted, but it became smaller in magnitude—about a thirteen-minute advantage for women.

"I was shocked," Dr. Burgard admitted to me. "The findings fly in the face of so much of what we know about men and women's roles in the home, and how women disproportionately take on the second and even third shifts in the home, referring to household responsibilities in general, as well as nighttime caregiving responsibilities, respectively."

But as she and her colleagues looked more closely at their data, it began to make sense. The largest gender gaps in sleep duration appeared during life stages in which caregiving responsibilities were highest (i.e., when respondents had children under the age of six in the home). Given that women disproportionately take on the nighttime caregiving activities for young children, this particular stage of life is also associated with high rates of interrupted sleep. In other words, women are sleeping a bit more in part to compensate for their lack of high-quality, uninterrupted sleep, especially when little ones are in the house. This also helps to reconcile the paradox between women's greater risk for sleep complaints and insomnia, despite having better objectively measured sleep (at least based on the current measurement approaches).

Quantity is certainly not the same thing as sleep quality. For women, our sleep, like many other aspects of our lives, is intricately entwined with the needs of others and with our connection to others. Women, if partnered and with the resources and flexibility to do so, may be able to compensate for interrupted sleep by going to bed earlier or napping. In contrast, Dr. Burgard's findings showed that men's sleep is largely constrained by work roles, both paid and unpaid, and was particularly pinched when young children were in the home. These are important findings as they suggest that although women's sleep quality may be more interrupted by nighttime caregiving activities for children, men's opportunity for sleep is reduced by the demands of both work hours and family responsibilities. In other words, it's important to recognize these potential differences and also acknowledge the unique challenges your partner may be experiencing with their sleep, which may be different from your own.

Although we frankly don't have the research on the challenges same-sex couples face in sleeping together (a research gap that needs to be filled), similar patterns may emerge as we see in heterosexual couples. However, it is important to note these biological sex differences in the prevalence of sleep disorders, as it may, for example, make male couples statistically more likely to have two snorers in a bed, whereas female couples may run a greater risk of having both partners with insomnia in the bed. Nevertheless, the same "rules" apply for same-sex and heterosexual couples: in both cases, recognizing your partner's sleep needs and challenges and how they jive or don't with yours is key to finding relationship harmony in that crucial third of our lives we spend asleep.

SHARED SLEEP ACTION PLAN:
Sleep Profiles

I find the research on gender differences in sleep fascinating, as it helps us get an even clearer picture of the many factors that influence our sleep as individuals and as couples. But for you and your shared bed, it's most important that you get a clear picture of your and your partner's sleep—to try to come to some sort of understanding about your individual habits and behaviors and how they might be affecting your or your partner's ability to get as healthy sleep as possible.

A great starting place to find this mutual ground and understanding with your partner is to talk about what's currently helping or hurting your sleep. What is your preferred method for winding down to prepare for a good night of sleep? This seems like a pretty obvious question that couples would naturally engage in, but in my experience it happens far too infrequently. Rather, the preferred method of winding down (or lack thereof) involves one partner basically taking over the bedroom, with the other partner unwittingly coming along for the ride. This happens a lot when it comes to technology use. I have seen many clients who bemoan that they simply can't relax and unwind before bed because their partner is typing away on their laptop or insists on having the TV on. I ask, "How did you all arrive at this arrangement?" And generally the response is, "I don't know. It just kind of happened. And now I feel like a nag to tell her to stop."

What constitutes relaxing activities for men and women also can differ. Perhaps the most salient example is sex. The general belief, despite the fact that there is really limited data on this topic in humans, is that sex is a soporific—it helps induce sleep. And that may be true for some. For others, however, sex can have the opposite effect—causing arousal, not in the sexual sense, but in the "now I can't fall asleep" sense. Some women reading this book might roll their eyes recalling all the times their partner fell fast asleep minutes after sex, leaving them sitting there ready to talk.

For this part of your shared sleep action plan, I want to help you and your partner start identifying your unique sleep profiles, from how you prefer to unwind, to the factors that may be helping or hurting your sleep, to any concerns you might have about possible sleep disorders. The profiles below guide you through a series of questions. Each partner should answer each question for themselves, independent of input from the other partner. Then, after you have completed the activity, share your responses to each question, and discuss how your individual profiles complement or sometimes conflict with each other. Next, together, identify some potential strategies you can put into practice that can help you find common ground in bed. If one partner watches TV to go to sleep and that keeps the other awake, perhaps you could try swapping the TV for some other wind-down activity. (Screens aren't good for sleep anyway.) If one partner wants to talk before falling asleep, and the other likes to lie quietly to wind down, perhaps you can go to bed a bit earlier so you can have your talk and the zone-out time.

Individual Sleep Profiles

Both you and your partner should answer these questions independently.

1. How well do you sleep? How much sleep do you get? Do you wake up feeling refreshed and ready to start your day? Are you concerned you may have a sleep disorder?
2. How well do you think your partner sleeps? Are you concerned he or she may have a sleep disorder?
3. Is there anything your partner does that affects your ability to sleep? If so, what is it?
4. If it were entirely up to you, what would be your ideal go-to-sleep scenario most nights. What would you do before going to bed? When would you go to bed? What would you do in bed? By when would you like to be asleep? When would you want to wake up?
5. How would you describe your sleep hygiene? Of the factors that are known to influence sleep, which may be positively or negatively affecting your ability to sleep as well as you'd like? What behaviors would you consider changing to improve your sleep?

Shared Action Plan

This part of the action plan should be completed with your partner.

1. Take some time to go through each of your responses to the individual sleep profiles with your partner, and discuss your similarities and differences.
2. After discussing your answers to each of the questions above, identify a shared sleep goal by discussing one thing you can both commit to trying this week to improve the quality of your sleep together. Maybe it's mutually agreeing to keep your phones out of the bedroom, or if that's too big a leap,

maybe it's simply setting a twenty- to thirty-minute window of tech-free time together before lights out. Or maybe you both want to work on being more consistent about your bedtimes and wake-up times. There are lots of ways to begin. Pick something achievable, and then write it down and keep your shared sleep goal in a place where you both can see it.

3. How might your relationship improve if you commit to your shared sleep goal?

4. At the end of the week, check in with each other. How successful were you in achieving your goal? If successful, what benefits, if any, did you see? If unsuccessful, what got in the way? What small tweaks could you make to be more successful? Maybe you were too ambitious about your goal. Remember, even small steps can make a big difference in sleep. Or maybe one or both of you wasn't really committed to pursuing this goal. If so, return to step 2.

chapter six

ROOM FOR MORE?

Penelope and Cyrus are in their early forties. They live in Cincinnati. Penelope is a university professor. Cyrus is an e-learning consultant for an education technology start-up. They have three kids—Oscar (age nine), Maya (age six), and Ruthie (age four). As Cyrus tells it, "We basically haven't had a good night's sleep for almost ten years. Those people who warned us about sleeping with kids weren't lying. When they're infants, it's hard. When they're toddlers, it's harder. And when there's three of them, it's impossible. Oscar didn't start sleeping through the night until he was four, but it didn't really help, because at that point one-year-old Maya was impossible to get down. And right when things were getting better with her, we went and had Ruthie! And as challenging as it was to sleep when Oscar and Maya were babies and toddlers, Ruthie has really taken it to the next level. We've tried sleep training, but we're terrible at it. We tried that whole cry-it-out thing. We were too wimpy to follow through with it. And at some point, I'm not sure when, we just gave up and decided to let Ruthie do what she wants. And what she wants is us. At this point, Ruthie is four, and every night around two a.m., she wakes up in her own bed. (We're able to get her to start there.) She then walks into our room and crawls into our bed and wedges herself in between Penelope and me and goes back to sleep. I try to sleep through it, but I can't sleep with a four-year-old sprawling out on me, so I then crawl out of our bed and go to Ruthie's room and into her bed. It's not made for a dude my size, but I attempt to sleep there every night! It only somewhat works. I asked Ruthie when she was going to spend the entire night in her own bed, and she said, 'When I'm thirteen.' I'm totally screwed."

Penelope and Cyrus have a good sense of humor about their situation, which helps, but they also both admit that their consistent lack of sleep for the last nine plus years has put a strain on all parts of their lives from their relationship, their parenting, their productivity at work, and their ability to simply maintain the household. Penelope says, "At this point, we're just waiting Ruthie out instead of trying to solve this problem, but I'm not sure how long we can wait. We're cranky. The house is pretty much always a disaster. I'm mailing it in at work. And I can't even sleep with my own husband. It's not good."

Penelope is right. It's not good. Unfortunately, theirs is also a very common experience for parents of small children. For many couples, the birth of their first child (not to mention the second, third, and so on) brings drama to the shared bed. From the time you bring that first little precious being home, your bed, presumably once a sacred space of respite and intimacy for you and your partner, is forever changed. If you keep bringing more kids home, as Cyrus and Penelope have done, the challenge just gets compounded. And of course, I'd like to reassure Cyrus and Penelope and all my readers that you can just wait them out, but as a parent of two teenagers, I can tell you, the sleeping challenges introduced when you first become a parent may wax and wane over your child's development, and morph in a variety of ways, but they don't just go away. Once you get beyond infancy and your child (one hopes) is sleeping through the night, then at about age three, many will see a spike in nightmares, which invites a whole new era of middle-of-the-night awakenings. Then there are the grade school years and the uptick in sleep problems that occurs for many children as they enter into kindergarten or start a new school. Jump ahead to the teenage years, and you can join me as I watch my adolescent children become ever more sleep-deprived as a result of the conflict between their early high school starting time and their sleep-wake biology, which favors later bedtimes and wake-up times.

Kids, as wonderful as they are, present challenges to your and your partner's ability to sleep individually and as a couple, but with a little proactive planning and communication, you and your partner can improve your sleep and your kids' sleep, which can improve a bunch of other things in the process.

TINY TORTURERS

In the wake of the 9/11 terrorist attacks, the US military engaged in a number of "enhanced interrogation techniques," including keeping prisoners awake for up to 180 hours as a means to produce actionable intelligence. Although there is ongoing debate as to whether sleep deprivation constitutes a form of torture, there is no question that prolonged sleep deprivation or random waking at all hours has profound effects on prisoners' ability to think clearly or act rationally, and it degrades their physical and mental health. It has also been shown to be ineffective, because the information provided by prisoners after such treatment tends to be less than reliable. We know that it's wrong to treat our prisoners of war this way, to make them wake up at random hours throughout the night, to deprive them of the mental and physical repair that sleep provides, but a lot of couples out there, at some point in their relationship, invite tiny yet powerful torturers into their homes and bedrooms.

Babies. They are so cute. They bring us so much joy, with their cooing and crawling and cuddling. But for all that our children bring to our lives, those first few years can literally feel a bit like torture. Just to be clear, I'm not really suggesting the sleep deprivation you and your partner experience when caring for your baby is anywhere close to the torture experienced by prisoners of war. However, the broken sleep parents with small children experience can have similar negative effects: it can hinder parents' ability to think clearly, to regulate mood, to maintain good health, and to stay productive. It's a slightly sadistic pastime of mine to hear couples' funny stories about the crazy things they did while in the throes of sleep deprivation as newborn parents (as long as they have happy endings), like the guy who used diaper cream instead of toothpaste on his toothbrush or my friend who went to work wearing a mismatched pair of shoes.

In my case, I knew I hit rock bottom when my son was nearly three and my daughter was just a few months old. I was driving to the Scientific Leadership and Management conference at the University of Pittsburgh (let that sink in once you hear the rest of this story), and I stopped to get gas on the way. As I pulled out of the gas station, I heard a loud *clunk* and saw several other customers staring at me and pointing, with their jaws dropped. In my sleep-starved haze, it took me a second to realize what I had done—I had driven away with the gas nozzle still connected to my car. I ripped the entire hose out of the tank. It's a miracle I didn't start an explosion. Luckily the attendant was very kind to me and let me go. He probably pitied me for being completely out of my mind. Then off I went, to be a "scientific leader," despite questionably functioning as an independent adult—thanks to sleep loss.

Even once we eventually get to a place where our kids aren't waking us at all hours and are sleeping in their own beds, the disruptions we experience in those early years can have lingering effects long after. This is why there's a whole subsection of self-help books dedicated to the various tips and tricks for sleep training your baby. And while it is important to help your child build good sleep habits, if you are in a couple, probably the best way for you to do that has less to do with which sleep training method you adopt (although some have more evidence behind them than others) and more to do with how you and your partner come together to create a shared plan around everyone's sleep—yours, your partner's, and your baby's. When you don't have such a shared plan, you can feel as if you're just stuck in a sleepless limbo until your baby finally reaches some mysterious developmental milestone that you can't predict or plan for. And that feeling of helplessness is painful and anxiety-provoking and can wreak havoc on your relationship.

In this chapter, I have no intention of taking a stance on how best to sleep train your baby. I know what I did with my kids, and I'll touch on some options so you have some exposure to the current wisdom out there. However, this book is about how you and your partner sleep as a couple. Getting your baby to sleep well will help with that, but you can read other books to get more specific guidance and strategies. Rather, I come to this part of the book with the basic recommendation that, as a couple, you need to mindfully, purposefully, and jointly discuss your family's values and the pros and cons of specific sleeping arrangements you want for yourselves and for your children. Upon doing so, you then need to come to a shared understanding of how you, as a couple, are going to manage sleeping as a family. That could lead you to select a specific sleep training strategy. It could also lead you somewhere else. The important thing is less about what you choose to do or not do and more about being on the same page about what you're doing. From this vantage point, you can then have healthy negotiations about what's working and what's not working with your given sleeping circumstances, and what can be done to ensure that both partners and your children are maximizing their opportunity for adequate sleep duration and good sleep quality. When you take steps to keep your own sleep a priority, even with the challenges that babies and toddlers and teenagers inflict on all that, you are taking steps to keep your relationship a priority as well. A well-slept partner is more likely to be a good partner! And that's what we're aiming for.

WHO DOES WHAT WHEN?

When your baby is an infant, there are two big questions related to your baby's nighttime needs, that you as a couple need to answer. First: How are you going to distribute labor when it comes to nighttime caregiving? Second: Where is this kid going to sleep? Let's start by looking at the first one, because if you and your partner can collaborate on a fair system for supporting each other as you support your infant's nighttime needs, it can lay the groundwork for open and honest communication about many other family-related sleep decisions.

So the big question couples need to answer is this: Who is going to go to baby Johnny when he wakes up crying, at one, three, and five in the morning (or some variation)? If partners don't collaborate to come up with a mutually agreed upon answer to this question, the resulting experience can bring out the worst in both of them, giving rise to major relationship strife. Sociologist Rob Meadows and colleagues at the University of Surrey have conducted elegant work focused on trying to better understand how couples negotiate the night and how gendered roles and expectations influence these decisions about nighttime caregiving activities. "What we found was most common when it came to discussions about the night were the silences, rather than overt discussion. Issues around nighttime caregiving for children were just assumed to be common sense. And often these assumptions were based on presumed biological 'givens,' such as the presumption that women are just more natural caregivers, and therefore should bear the brunt of the nighttime caregiving responsibilities." A major takeaway from this work, according to Dr. Meadows, was "Don't default to this idea of what is 'natural' or 'biological.' That's really just a strategy to reduce a complex issue that ideally requires open and honest communication to an overly simplified solution, that may ultimately breed resentment and hostility."

It's also important to note that, even though men and women may experience sleep and sleep disruption differently, research shows that in many couples the burden of sleep deprivation is felt by both moms and dads. In one study, mothers of infants actually obtained more sleep than fathers. But before you dads out there go around saying "I told you so," they also found that mothers' sleep was more disturbed. So even though mothers logged more total hours, they were more likely to experience the torture of repeatedly broken sleep. What's worse is that for mothers, the disrupted sleep patterns and associated consequences on daytime functioning (like sleepiness, fatigue, cognitive impairments) persist even after the baby starts sleeping through the night. In other words, "mommy brain"—that spacy, sleep-deprived state when moms feel as if their brains are in a fog and can't think straight—is a real thing, and it doesn't just go away once the baby starts sleeping through the night. In fact, research has shown that nearly half of moms experienced moderate to severe daytime sleepiness, even when their baby reached age two and a half. All these broken nights of sleep add up over time and can lead to a very wobbly new mom.

I say this not as a scare tactic to discourage anyone from the many, many joys of parenthood, but as a wake-up call for couples to recognize how important it is to support each other both day and night as you enter parenthood. Being sleep-deprived can make you pretty miserable to be around and a not-so-pleasant partner, and it can profoundly affect your mental health. Studies show that mothers with disturbed sleep have increased rates of depressive symptoms and clinically significant postpartum depression, as well as higher parenting stress, and poorer maternal-infant bonding and sensitivity. Of course, since the beginning of time, sleep deprivation among new parents has been a fact of life, so while it is "natural" to be sleep-deprived after the birth of your child, I want to harken back to Dr. Meadows's words that just because something is "natural" doesn't mean we have to passively sit by and suffer the consequences, particularly when, for some, sleep deprivation can lead to long-term consequences for their mental health and the quality of their relationship.

Luckily, there is something you can do about it. Here are a few dos and don'ts for new parents to avoid letting sleep deprivation cause lasting harm to their relationship:

1. **Rally your support system so you have the opportunity to nap, and if the opportunity is there, then take it!** For example, promising evidence suggests that paying back sleep debt via scheduled naps could be beneficial for mother and child. Research has shown that taking a thirty- to forty-minute nap can counteract the negative effects of sleep deprivation. Research has also shown that mothers who took more frequent naps demonstrated more positive interactions with their children. In another study, mothers who napped less than sixty minutes during the day were at significantly increased risk for depression at three months postpartum. Importantly, these studies in mothers were all observational studies, so they cannot show that there is a causal link between napping and maternal behavior and well-being. In other words, it's possible that what's really driving the benefit is that mothers who choose to nap, or more importantly, have the opportunity to nap, have access to resources, including a supportive partner, family members, or friends who make it possible to take a nap. In fact, if there is one gift you could give to your partner or a friend or family member who has recently had a baby, offer to come over so they can take a nap! Forgo the chitchat and coffee; just let the poor parent go to sleep. Unfortunately, I think this is yet another reflection of our culture's tendency to undermine the importance of sleep. Rather than give new parents the gift they need most of all (which is to sleep), we have all of these socially proscribed patterns that often force

new parents into feeling they have to entertain visiting family and friends who come to meet the baby. As the saying goes, it does take a village to support healthy couples and happy families, and as part of that village, we should all do our part to support the sleep of new parents, as it is truly a foundation of health, well-being, and successful parenthood. Partners can be an important resource here—both to provide opportunities for each other to nap and to encourage each other, if Aunt Sally stops by to see the baby, let her do just that. Avoid the social pressure to entertain, and go take a nap together!

2. **Use caffeine wisely and judiciously.** Caffeine is the most widely consumed drug, and there's good reason—it works. Breastfeeding moms should exercise some caution and avoid large quantities of caffeine (e.g., in the form of energy pills or other stimulants, or highly caffeinated energy drinks). However, a well-timed cup of coffee—about an hour after waking in the morning—can give you an energy boost that can at least partially mitigate the pain of those sleepless nights. You can time your caffeine consumption to occur after breastfeeding or pumping in the morning. And it's always a good idea to talk to your pediatrician or other health care provider about any concerns about the impact of caffeine consumption on your breastfeeding baby. But my feeling is there are risks and benefits to just about everything, and we need to carefully balance the risk associated with feeling like a zombie all the time (one of which may be lashing out at your partner) versus having a cup of joe (which may require you to give up breastfeeding).

3. **Don't ever assume your partner had a good night of sleep just because you did.** Remember that even though mothers

and fathers of infants log about the same total amount of sleep, mothers fare worse when it comes to waking up throughout the night. Therefore, take this note of warning from my dear friend Laura, mother of twin girls, who shared that her husband's biggest mistake was when he would occasionally wake up after a night of sleep and say to her, "Wow. I can't believe the girls slept through the night." Nothing can evoke a mother's rage more than her partner's apparent obliviousness to the numerous awakenings that he was lucky enough not to hear. Always ask; don't assume it was a good night simply because it was for you.

4. **Talk about a healthy and fair division of labor — recognizing both partners' needs and schedules.** Don't fall into the trap shown by the majority of parents interviewed in the study by Dr. Meadows and colleagues that the most common approach to dividing nighttime caregiving responsibilities is to say nothing at all. Couples should talk about strategies to balance each other's sleep needs and daytime demands. Obviously, particularly if one parent is breastfeeding, there are some very real physical limitations that may require more of her involvement than the other parent's, but partners can help by taking on a nighttime feeding using expressed milk. This was a crucial strategy for my sanity with both of my babies. My husband and I had a strategy in which I would breastfeed the baby around nine p.m., then promptly take myself to bed. He would take on the midnight feeding using a bottle with milk I had pumped previously. Honestly, it was a game changer for me, to just be able to get that solid chunk of five to six hours of sleep before I would take on the next feeding, around three a.m. It was also a special and

important time for my husband, as the non-breastfeeding parent can sometimes feel pushed aside and struggle to find their own bond with the baby. Having open, honest, and strategic conversations about who's doing what at night is particularly important if both parents are returning to work. Ideally, some give and take is needed so each parent can get a break from the sleep deprivation on a regular basis, to avoid the cumulative build-up of sleep debt. But don't have these conversations late at night (or worse yet in the middle of the night), when you will be at your worst in terms of communication and problem-solving skills. Plan in advance, and set reasonable expectations of each other.

5. **Consider separate sleeping arrangements on occasion, so that at least one of you gets a solid night of sleep.** Part of that balancing act of giving each other the opportunity to get a solid night of sleep every once in a while might involve letting your partner sleep in a separate bedroom on occasion, if you happen to have the space. Maybe your partner has an important work meeting coming up, or maybe they are becoming emotionally frayed and just need to sleep. Give them the gift of allowing them to sleep in a separate bedroom while you take on the overnight responsibilities. Consider it a sleep vacation from each other. Pay it forward, and know that when you need it, your partner will do the same.

WHERE WILL THE BABY SLEEP?

How you manage the work of helping the baby (and yourselves) sleep is one big set of decisions for any couple. Another key question you need to answer is where your precious infant will sleep. Many of us look to our friends, our parents, and medical experts to inform this critically important family decision, but the result is often a tangle of incompatible and complicated to understand advice. The current guidance from the American Academy of Pediatrics states, "It is recommended that infants sleep in the parents' room, close to the parents' bed, but on a separate surface designed for infants, ideally for the first year of life, but at least for the first 6 months." Kind of a mouthful, right? The guidance suggests that parents can bring their baby into bed for a feeding or for soothing, but should return the baby to their own bed once they are fed or soothed.

This guidance is based on evidence that shows this type of sleeping arrangement is the best safeguard against sudden infant death syndrome, or SIDS—every parent's worst nightmare. The problem is that the guidance is sort of hard to understand and, almost inevitably, hard to follow to the letter and can lead to feelings of guilt or shame when we inevitably deviate from the recommendations. For example, a breastfeeding mom who unintentionally falls asleep in bed with her infant, a high-probability scenario given that she is sleep-deprived, essentially is being told that she gets an F on her parenting report card. Even though she followed the recommendation to breastfeed, that's cancelled out because she fell asleep with her child in her bed. And the truth is that many families (45 percent or more), at least some of the time, co-sleep with their infants—meaning they just bring the baby into their bed with them throughout the entire night. These are not bad parents, but many parents who make this very reasonable decision can be left feeling closeted and shamed, particularly when speaking to their pediatrician, who should otherwise be someone they can turn to openly and honestly with questions and concerns about their infants' sleep needs, without fear of judgment.

When I had my own children, my husband and I started with the idea that we were going to co-sleep. This decision was largely based on my upbringing, as I was raised by parents who were firm believers in attachment parenting, which aims to promote parent-infant bonding through warmth and responsiveness and through high levels of physical contact and intimacy, including co-sleeping. A substantial amount of research supports the benefits of attachment parenting, and I figured, "Well, I turned out alright," so we thought we'd give it a whirl. And at least initially, my husband was onboard, but in the end it just didn't work for either of us. None of us was sleeping well, our relationship was suffering, and I was feeling a whole lot of guilt. It took a long time for my husband and me to talk through our own expectations and beliefs about co-sleeping, and about the reality of the co-sleeping relationship for us, before we could arrive at a decision that worked for our family. Ultimately, we opted for a bassinet in our bedroom for about the first six months of our children's lives and then moved them to a crib in their own bedroom after six months. Unfortunately, too often couples bypass the conversation about their values, goals, and practical concerns and make decisions out of sleep-deprived desperation, without thinking about the downstream effects.

As much as I do not have objections to co-sleeping and think that for some families it can absolutely be the right choice for them, I think it's important to remember that infants, like full-grown adults, are creatures of habit. Therefore, if the habit is for the child to snuggle up in bed with their parents, then it is unfair to think that when the parents wake up one day and decide they've had enough of this situation, the little one will magically march to their own room and happily and peacefully fall asleep in their own bed. It's more than habit, too: recall that sleep is evolutionarily a vulnerable state to be in—especially for infants and children. A child's desire to sleep with their parents is totally natural. But just because it's natural doesn't mean it will work for everyone. This is one of the many hard parts of being a parent. It's about recognizing that the child's needs in this case may be incompatible with the parents' needs. By recognizing this conflict, parents can be sensitive and nurturing to their children while at the same time responsive to their own needs.

Also keep in mind one of the defining features of early childhood: almost everything changes at some point. When you catch yourself worrying whether you are going to have this child sleeping in a starfish position in between you and your partner for the rest of your lives, I'm here to tell you, that is very unlikely. If getting your child out of your bed is your goal, then there are ways to do it that don't involve letting your child cry it out for hours on end. In fact, one of the most recommended and evidence-based treatments for helping children to sleep independently is called "graduated extinction." In this approach, parents start in the desired sleep location with their child (e.g., in the child's room, standing next to the crib) and gradually, over successive nights or sometimes weeks, move further away from the child and eventually out of the room.

I'll be honest that with my daughter, this was somewhat of a protracted process, and it was actually several months before I could walk out of her room and just go about my evening. For longer than I care to admit, I would sit on the floor outside her room, until eventually she became comfortable enough to hear me walk down the stairs and away from the room. I was okay with this. And of course, it helped that my husband did his fair share of sitting outside the door as well. For my husband and me, this strategy balanced our desire to have our child sleep independently with her fundamental need for safety and security at night. By taking it very gradually, we were able to meet all of our needs.

The problem for many couples is that the decision to co-sleep or not is not a mutual one. Research shows that when couples are not on the same page when it comes to their infants' sleeping arrangements, this can be both a cause and a consequence of problems in the couples' relationship dynamic. For example, research has shown that relationship dissatisfaction in the parents predicted the infant's sleeping arrangement at six months of age. Specifically, when mothers who co-slept with their infants at one month of age reported high levels of relationship dissatisfaction with their partners, they were more likely to continue to co-sleep with their infants by six months of age. In contrast, when mothers who co-slept at one month reported they had a good relationship with their partner, they were more likely to move their infants into solitary sleep arrangements by six months. When the researchers looked at the reverse association (whether infant sleeping arrangements predict changes in parent relationship satisfaction), they found absolutely no association. This finding suggests that it is less about the baby driving a wedge in your relationship; rather, if you don't attend to issues in your relationship, it can manifest in sleeping arrangements that may not work for one or both parents. A primary task, therefore, of coparenting couples is to be explicit about what their own expectations are for infant sleep arrangements, including recognition of how their own family and sociocultural makeup has influenced these expectations.

As a working parent myself, I empathize deeply with the working parents who feel that co-sleeping is the one time for quality and extended time with their infant. I also empathize with their partners, who, like my own, may not feel the same need to co-sleep or, even if they do, may feel a stronger need to protect their intimate time in bed with their partner alone.

For example, Casey and Alex came to me with concerns about their one-year-old daughter's sleep. At the beginning of our initial evaluation, I asked both parents, "What is your goal for this treatment?" Casey answered, "To get Lily to sleep through the night." Alex, on the other hand, answered, "To get Lily to sleep through the night in her own room." Just four words ("in her own room") distinguished their goals, but within those four words lay the source of great conflict and increasing estrangement between Casey and Alex. Neither partner felt their concerns or needs were being heard, and neither felt that their needs for sleep or closeness were being met. In therapy, we worked on helping both partners communicate their concerns. Casey feared "irreparable" harm to Lily if they let her cry it out—which, by the way, is not the only or even the recommended strategy to sleep train infants these days. Alex feared that they would never return to their former shared couple bed, without the intrusion of a child. My work with them as well as many other couples facing similar challenges involved helping them to communicate their sleep and intimacy needs, as well as their beliefs, values, and concerns about infant co-sleeping. For some, this means challenging the notion that a shared bedroom or bed is an essential part of romantic partnership. For others, however, keeping the bedroom as a sacred space for the couple is critical for maintaining intimacy and connection between the partners.

SHARED SLEEP ACTION PLAN:
Sleeping Together (with a Baby!)

A key message from this chapter is that how you manage your baby's sleep needs is less important than making sure you and your partner have come to that "how" through shared decision making. Taking time to make sure you have talked through things like where the baby will sleep, what your goals are for everyone's (your, your partner's, and the baby's) sleep, how you will share duties throughout the night, and more can help make it easier for everyone to weather the sleepless storm that rolls in with your baby. For this installment of your Shared Sleep Action Plan, connect with your partner and talk through the following questions, making sure you each answer every question from your personal perspectives. Simply taking time to discuss these questions can go a long way to establishing that mutual understanding that is so critical for successfully weathering the challenges of new parenthood and even strengthening your relationship along the way.

> **Question 1:** What is your priority when it comes to your and your baby's sleep and why? For example, is your goal to help your infant self-soothe and sleep independently as quickly as possible? Are you seeking sleep as an opportunity to bond with your baby at night? Do you want to do whatever you can to make sure your sleep is prioritized above all else? Remember just a few words can make a difference in your goals, so be explicit in what you want and why.
>
> **Question 2:** Are you satisfied with your and your child's current sleeping arrangements? If yes, why? If not, why?

Question 3: What assumptions about sleep and babies do you bring based on your own upbringing, cultural background, or exposure to other people with babies? What did your parents do with you or your siblings? (If you don't know, you might ask them, if that's possible.)

Question 4: How can you best support each other's sleep needs while supporting a baby's needs throughout the night? What are you willing to do for each other to make sure you both get as much sleep as possible? How can you get creative?

Question 5: What sleep training methods do you know about or have you tried? What worked or hasn't worked about the particular method(s) you've tried? What additional resources could you engage to help you achieve your goals? For example, you could read a book on sleep training. Or you could hire a sleep consultant.

chapter seven

ARE WE IN SYNC?

TERESA WAS BORN IN PUERTO RICO AND IMMIGRATED TO THE United States in her teens. Throughout her life, Teresa was an extreme night owl. Her high school years were particularly brutal, because she felt her most alert and creative in the late evening hours, making it virtually impossible for her to fall asleep before two a.m. and rendering her a total zombie when she had to wake up for school at six thirty a.m. Although she was not alone in struggling to get enough sleep, because most teenagers show a biologically driven "phase delay" (meaning a preference for later bedtimes and later wake-up times) during that stage of development, she had a phase delay that wasn't just restricted to her adolescence. With persistence, she managed to get through high school, followed by college and a master's degree in education, though she notes that those high school years of chronic sleep deprivation nearly killed her.

A natural educator, Teresa started her career as a teacher and worked her way up to an administrative role in an urban school district. In the context of her chosen profession, her night-owl tendencies did have some advantages. Because the work of a teacher or administrator is seemingly never done, it was not a problem for her to stay up into the wee hours working. Mornings, on the other hand, continued to be brutal. But by that point in her life, she had just accepted the painful early wake-up woes as a fact of her life.

Teresa met her husband, John, an engineer, when they were both in their thirties. They connected with each other through their love of books, the outdoors, and travel. John loved Teresa's free-spirited, passionate personality and her seemingly endless supply of energy. Teresa fell in love with John's kind-heartedness, stability, and great sense of humor. Ironically, they first met in a bar on a night when it was way past John's usual bedtime. He was (and is) Teresa's polar opposite when it comes to his preferred sleep and wake schedule. They often joked that it was a miracle they even met. Even in his bachelor days, it was a struggle for John to stay out after eleven p.m. Teresa, on the other hand, often found herself salsa dancing until two a.m. John did his best work and thinking in the early morning: he had a regular rise time of five a.m. and a bedtime of ten p.m. Teresa's mind and body wouldn't allow her to go to sleep so early. As a loving, compromising couple, they both tried to accommodate the other.

For many years, John tried to adapt to Teresa's owl schedule by forcing himself to stay up later than his usual ten p.m. bedtime. For her part, Teresa would get in bed with him far earlier than she was ready to (albeit with laptop in hand). It wasn't a perfect situation, but they both felt it was a necessary compromise for the sake of their relationship. It took its toll on both of them, but particularly on Teresa, as trying to force herself to fall asleep hours before her natural clock was ready for sleep resulted in a pattern of not being able to fall asleep, followed by frustration, leading to even greater difficulty falling asleep, which is a classic cycle of insomnia.

The situation took a turn for the worse when Teresa retired. Without the requirement of her work schedule, Teresa's natural sleep-wake rhythm drifted even later. John, who was still working, was not pleased. Even without the demands of work, Teresa was still highly involved in community service work and other creative projects, which she continued to work on in bed. John felt that Teresa should be the one to compromise for his schedule because he was still working and was getting more and more fed up with hearing the *tap, tap* of her keyboard as he tried to fall asleep at night. Teresa, on the other hand, was feeling judged and invalidated. It painfully brought her back to her high school days, when she felt as if all of the adults in her life—her parents, teachers, and coaches—ascribed her inability to sleep at a reasonable hour and her chronic daytime sleepiness as a sign of laziness or poor self-regulation, rather than the intrinsic rhythm of her body. To make matters worse, the years of insomnia were deeply affecting her, because she found that rather than enjoying the freedom of her retirement, she was feeling increasingly irritable, anxious, and sleep-deprived. Her days were now filled with worries about whether she would be able to fall asleep the subsequent night. With the build-up of those negative emotions came resentment, specifically directed toward John.

UNDERSTANDING YOUR OWN AND
YOUR PARTNER'S CHRONOTYPE

Some people are owls. They hit their stride late into the evening hours. Others are larks. They wake up cheerfully at the crack of dawn. In the United States, larks have a natural advantage over owls. We live in a society that tends to view morningness as a virtue. We cast shame on the "lazy" evening types who just can't seem to get it together to go to bed (or wake up) at a reasonable time. The truth of the matter is that our preferences for morningness or eveningness, otherwise known as chronotype, are largely hardwired in our DNA. About 50 percent of the variability is accounted for by genetics, while other factors, like age and gender, also play a role.

Chronotypes are typically measured by scales that reflect a continuum representing peak times of alertness and optimal functioning throughout the day. While extreme larks and owls are found at the tails of this continuum, the majority of the population are "third birds," falling somewhere in the middle. A quick way of determining your chronotype is to calculate your preferred midpoint of sleep on a free day—that is, a nonworking day, or a day you don't have to wake up to an alarm. To do so, calculate your average sleep duration, divide that number by two, then add the outcome to your preferred bedtime. For example, if your average weekend bedtime is midnight and you wake up at eight a.m., your sleep midpoint is four a.m. (midnight + four hours).

About 60 percent of us have sleep midpoints between three thirty a.m. and five a.m.—we are the third birds. Note that your preferred midpoint on your free days could be quite different from your sleep pattern or midpoint during the week. For those who tend towards the owl side of the spectrum, this can be particularly challenging, because external demands like work or school schedules or family responsibilities force you to be awake and asleep at times that are inconsistent with your internal rhythms. Chronobiologist Dr. Till Roenneberg has termed this phenomenon "social jetlag": when your sleep midpoint on weekdays is two or more hours different (usually later) than your sleep midpoint on nonfree days. Just look at a teenager if you ever want to see what social jetlag looks like. Monday through Friday, teenagers have to go to school at inhumanely early hours (most US high schools start at or before eight a.m.), despite the fact that during adolescence there is a known biological shift towards eveningness, which is specific to that developmental period. In the context of couples, and given our cultural favoritism toward morning types, if one member is a lark and the other an owl, this can set the stage for disharmony in the nest. No matter how much nagging, cajoling, and berating you may try, it's a tall order to override someone's biological clock.

What many people do not realize, including Teresa and John, is that not only are our circadian rhythms hardwired, but they also govern more than just when we feel most awake and when we feel most sleepy. Science shows us that we all have little clocks inside of virtually every cell in our body. These clocks regulate a broad range of behaviors and physiology, including our moods, hunger, productivity and sex drive, and even our blood pressure or when our cells die or proliferate (which is one of the reasons why circadian rhythms and sleep are currently hot topics in cancer research). We all also have one central master clock that is located in our brains, in an area of the hypothalamus known as the suprachiasmatic nucleus. This master clock is supposed to keep all of the other little clocks throughout the body in sync and running on roughly a twenty-four-hour rhythm. To be more precise, it's twenty-four hours and eleven minutes, on average, which makes sense, because the word "circadian" literally translates as "about a day." As many of us have experienced—with jet lag, for example—sometimes our central clock and our peripheral clocks get a bit out of whack, making us feel hungry or sleepy at the "wrong" times of day. Or it can make us simply feel all around crummy until our body eventually shifts back into sync after a few days on the new schedule. But for people consistently living out of sync with their internal rhythms (like Teresa), the fatigue, malaise, and all-around crumminess can be more enduring.

There are known sex and individual differences in when and how long our clocks run. For example, there is a greater likelihood for women to prefer earlier bedtimes and earlier rise times. Women are more likely than men to be morning larks. Studies have also shown that women show a stronger preference for activity earlier in the day than men. Women's clocks also run up to a full six minutes shorter, meaning that a woman's "day" is crammed into a shorter period than men's. No wonder "a woman's work is never done." We simply have less time to do it!

Of course, these are broad generalities, but in addition to sex differences, there are also variations in circadian rhythms at the individual level, as in the Teresa and John example. In Teresa's case, although she came to me with insomnia (which by that point she definitely had), it turned out that the root of her problem was that she had delayed sleep phase syndrome, or DSPS. This disorder, which afflicts about four hundred thousand Americans, is more than just being a night owl. People with DSPS literally can't fall asleep earlier even if they want to because their circadian rhythms are delayed by at least two hours (and often much more) than the typical rhythm. For Teresa, that meant that try as hard as she might to go to bed even by midnight, both to appease her husband and to allow for getting at least six hours of sleep (still well under the recommended seven to eight hours sleep duration), she often wouldn't be able to fall asleep until two a.m. What's truly remarkable about Teresa, like the many other people living with DSPS, is that she managed to not only keep her job but excel as a school teacher and administrator. Monday through Friday, she forced her body to align with society's schedule, which was out of sync with her own internal rhythm, resulting in chronic sleep deprivation, not to mention all of the other unpleasant effects of jet lag, like malaise, daytime sleepiness, moodiness, and more.

In my work with Teresa, the first step was giving her a name for what she had been experiencing all of her life. DSPS was why she struggled so terribly with waking up in the mornings or going to bed at a "reasonable" hour. It was not just a lack of willpower or self-regulation. This validation was incredibly powerful for her because over time she had internalized the negative judgments that she had been receiving throughout her life, including from her husband. The next step was helping Teresa communicate with John that her late-night proclivities weren't merely her personal choice but rather a hardwired predisposition. Working with them as a couple, I also helped them both understand that throughout the day, their different rhythms affect more than just when they felt sleepy. They also affect many other critical aspects of their relationship functioning, ranging from when they feel most alert and happy to when they are best able to communicate and problem solve and when they are most likely to enjoy sex. The problem for many couples like Teresa and John is that they regularly engage in inherent tasks of partnership, like having disagreements, but they do so at a time of day that, for at least one partner, was at their low point of effective communication and problem-solving skills.

For Teresa and John, their mutual frustrations over John's demands for an early bedtime and Teresa's practice of bringing her computer into bed led to disagreements in the evening hours, a time that was far from optimal for John's lark tendencies. The work for them was to discover how they could honor and respect each of their rhythms and needs, while finding some mutually agreeable time of day to enjoy each other's company and allow both partners an opportunity for good quality sleep. Ultimately, this involved carving out quality time for them to share together in the early evening hours, before John went to bed, so that they could just be together and, if necessary, deal with whatever hot topics may have arisen in their relationship. As much as possible, avoiding heavy discussions after nine p.m. was an important step for them because even John recognized that he couldn't think clearly, let alone be rational and open to compromise, once he got too sleepy. For Teresa, even though they lived in a small apartment, part of the process of helping her feel more validated was finding her the physical space she needed to engage in her creative projects at night, but not in bed. They chose the dining room table, which was rarely used, but just what Teresa needed to feel that her needs and her natural tendency to feel creative at night were respected and valued.

Teresa and John are not alone in their struggles emanating from their different circadian rhythms. Research has shown that couples who are mismatched in their sleep-wake preferences show lower levels of relationship satisfaction, experience greater conflict, and have less sex. Importantly, however, most of this research is cross-sectional, so it is not clear whether differences in sleep-wake preferences lead to relationship distress, or whether relationship distress drives couples toward more divergent sleep-wake patterns, as a means to avoid the offending partner. However, research that my colleagues and I have conducted has shown that couples who are more in sync with their sleep do enjoy some relationship advantages.

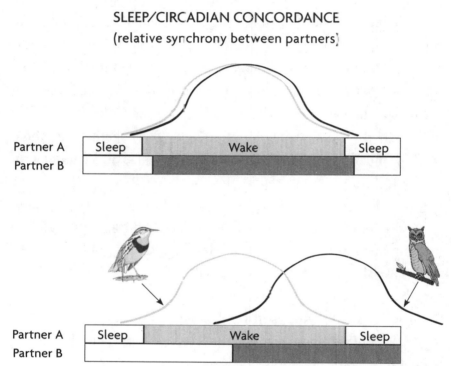

SLEEP/CIRCADIAN CONCORDANCE
(relative synchrony between partners)

In the upper panel, you see a couple (Partner A and B) who are nearly perfectly in sync with their sleep-wake rhythms, in that they share the same sleep and wake periods. The lower panel shows an example of a mismatched pair's sleep-wake schedule. In this case, Partner A is a morning lark who goes to bed early and wakes up early, whereas Partner B is a night owl, whose bedtimes and wake-up times are both shifted later. As you can see from this mismatched pair, they have considerably less time shared together when they are both awake or asleep. *Figure courtesy of Dr. Brant Hasler.*

In one study, led by Dr. Heather Gunn, we measured the sleep patterns of couples on a minute-to-minute basis throughout the night.

We found that those who were asleep or awake at the same times were more satisfied in their relationships. In a subsequent study, we found that couples who were more in sync also showed lower levels of an important marker of inflammation, called C-reactive protein, which has been associated with heart disease risk. These findings are among the first to suggest a direct physiological benefit of co-sleeping for adults. Of course, the benefits are likely contingent on whether both partners are sleeping well. In another study, we found that on nights when couples go to bed at the same time, women reported better relationship satisfaction the next day. Although we did not find the same effect for men, the findings do suggest that the behavioral act of going to bed together may help to fulfill one or both partner's needs for closeness and connection, even if the couple doesn't ultimately sleep together.

Now before all you mismatched pairs run off in despair, there is hope. Research also shows that couples who are mismatched in their sleep/wake patterns, but who have good problem-solving skills, are able to overcome the challenges otherwise associated with being out of sync. This is an important take-home message, because for many couples it's not about a mismatch in intrinsic schedules but rather extrinsic demands (e.g., work schedules) that lead to divergent schedules.

SYNCING UP WITH A SHIFT WORKER

Suzy and Peter are both physicians. They have been married for nineteen years and have two young children. She is in family medicine, and he is in emergency medicine. As an ER doctor who works on a rotating shift schedule, about one-third of the time working nights, Peter joins the roughly fifteen million Americans who work nights or "graveyard" shifts (typically eleven p.m. to seven a.m.). The challenge for Peter and his family is that because he is on a rotating schedule, meaning that week to week he may shift from working days to working nights, he never can fully adjust his sleep-wake pattern to any schedule. Whether working days or nights, he is almost always out-of-sync with the rhythm of the rest of his family, and he is always sleep-deprived.

As Suzy described it, managing Peter's sleep and how it fits in (or really doesn't fit in) with the rest of the family is a major focus of the family dynamic. "It's huge. The hardest part is, honestly, the mornings, when he is working nights and so he tries to sleep downstairs after returning from his shift at five or six a.m. He's trying to sleep, and I'm trying to get the kids out the door, but it's doubly stressful, because I have to rush them around the house while trying to make them as quiet as possible. It makes me superstressed, because the stakes are really high for our family. If Peter doesn't get good sleep, it affects how he interacts with us. It affects his patients. It affects his health. It even affects his safety on the road coming home. Thinking about him driving home after a long night shift, when I know he has not been sleeping well during the days, definitely can keep me up at night." She's not wrong about being concerned for his safety. Physicians and other medical workers routinely top the list for occupations with some of the highest rates of motor vehicle accidents.

Beyond the stress of the mornings, and the toll that Peter's chronic sleep deprivation takes on all of them, Suzy also acknowledged that his schedule has been the major challenge they've faced as a couple. "We just sort of lack that sense of normalcy—that daily routine of touching base, that most couples get when you return from work in the evenings. So if we have a free night, on the one hand, we feel this sense of obligation to go out and do something 'special,' but there's this other part of us that just needs to emotionally connect, regroup, and talk about all the usual family stuff, that we don't have time to do when we are operating on entirely different schedules. It's like you constantly feel like you are playing catch-up. That's the rhythm of our life right now."

The real solution for Peter and Suzy's situation, and the many other couples in which one or both members work shifts, is that we need some policy-level changes, including restricting the length of shifts and ensuring better scheduling, so that employees who have to rotate between days and nights are given sufficient time for recovery sleep and to adjust their sleep schedules from days to nights. Unfortunately, part of our cultural tendency to undermine the importance of sleep (to our own detriment) is reflected in the resistance to making reasonable regulations on shift-work schedules in a variety of industries, from medicine to transportation. Short of these necessary policy-level changes, there are several things couples can do to find some common ground, whether rhythms are out of sync because of intrinsic differences in sleep-wake schedules or external demands like work schedules.

1. **Become aware of your own and your partner's rhythms.** Use the Shared Sleep Action Plan at the end of this chapter to help each of you identify whether you are more of a lark or more of an owl. You can calculate each of your own scores, then subtract the two scores to find out how discrepant you are from each other in your natural rhythms. The bigger the discrepancy, the more problem solving you will both need to do to try to pinpoint what period of the day is going to be optimal for both of you to engage in pleasurable activities, to

be intimate, or to have those heavy, perhaps conflict-prone conversations.

2. **Respect each other's right to sleep.** This may mean that if your partner is a night owl or has to work night shifts, they may not be able to go to sleep at the same time you do and may function best if they can sleep in later (provided that work schedules can also be flexible). Try to use this discrepancy as a resource in your family, rather than a sticking point. For example, if you have young children in the home, and if one of you is more of a night person than the other, use that to your advantage. Have the night owl take on the evening child care responsibilities.

3. **Savor the time and space before falling asleep.** For many couples, it is the time before falling asleep that is most critical for a healthy and happy relationship. Even if you have different sleep-wake patterns or sleep in separate bedrooms, preserve that time together before you fall asleep, and use the time to be together, to connect, cuddle, or talk. Avoid engaging in activities like both of you individually watching Netflix or scrolling through emails. These activities are decidedly not relationship-enhancing or sleep-promoting. For example, if you are an owl and your partner is a lark, you could spend some time together in bed before your partner falls asleep, then quietly leave the room, and return at your more natural, later bedtime. Your partner can even try using an eye mask or ear plugs to reduce the likelihood that your return to bed will wake them up. In the mornings, your partner can start their early bird day and return later to wish you good morning, ideally with coffee in hand.

One could draw the conclusion from this chapter that if you are actively in search of a relationship, you might want to consider chronotype as an important factor for your next partner, and there is some wisdom in that. Understanding your partner (or future partner's) chronotype is important, because chronotype has a big influence on our moods, our functioning, our productivity, and how we spend our time. And yet you would be hard-pressed to find an online dating site that incorporates chronotype into their profile analysis. Nevertheless, it is something to consider because it can have a big impact on your relationship. That said, I wouldn't go so far as to say it should be a mate selection factor. Sometimes having complementary characteristics in a couple can be a real strength, if the couple uses it to their advantage. For example, if little ones are in the picture, and one partner is a night owl and the other a lark, the owl could take on some of the nighttime caregiving responsibilities, while the lark steps in for the early morning hours. In general, we shouldn't look for our clones in a partner, but rather someone who shares some of our values, likes, and dislikes but also brings something new to the table, so that we can complement each other's personality. At the same time, we have to acknowledge our differences, particularly when they are hardwired like sleep-wake preferences, and find ways to problem solve and negotiate the day *and* night with our partner.

SHARED SLEEP ACTION PLAN:
Assessing Your Synchronicity (or Lack of It)

Understanding how aligned or misaligned your and your partner's sleep rhythms are can go a long way in your collective effort to improve sleep for both of you. For this part of your Shared Sleep Action Plan, you and your partner should each take the assessment and then follow the instructions for scoring it. The assessment will help you each determine your individual chronotypes. It will also help you determine if and by how much you differ. Having that information can help you better craft a shared strategy for making sure you both get the sleep you need when you need it while also tending to other critical aspects of your relationship.

Directions: Both you and you partner can complete this scale. For each item, check one response that best describes you. To find your sleep-wake preference, add up your total score for all thirteen items based on the number in parentheses for each item you check. If you score 44 or higher, you are a morning type, with really high scores indicating an even stronger preference for mornings. If you score between 23 and 43, you are a third bird, meaning you don't have a particularly strong inclination toward morningness or eveningness. If you score a 22 or less, you are an evening type; the lower the score, the more strongly evening type you are. Once you and your partner have tallied up your scores, use them as an opportunity to investigate how matched or mismatched you are in your rhythms. Are you a lark (score of 44 or more) and your partner a third bird (score of 23–43) or perhaps an owl (<22)? If so, how does this play out in your relationship? Whose schedule do you follow, or do you follow separate schedules? Is this working for you both? Even if you are both in the same category of "bird," if one of you is on the upper end of the range and the other is on the lower end, this is an important opportunity for you to discuss how your schedules, both independent and shared, are working or not working for you both and to identify your prime times as a couple to engage in important couple activities, like being intimate, having fun together, or discussing hot topics.

COMPOSITE MORNINGNESS QUESTIONNAIRE

1. Considering only your own "feeling best" rhythm, at what time would you get up if you were entirely free to plan your day?

    ___ 5:00–6:30 a.m. (5)
    ___ 6:30–7:45 a.m. (4)
    ___ 7:45–9:45 a.m. (3)
    ___ 9:45–11:00 a.m. (2)
    ___ 11:00 a.m.–12:00 noon (1)

2. Considering only your own "feeling best" rhythm, at what time would you go to bed if you were entirely free to plan your evening?

    ___ 8:00–9:00 p.m. (5)
    ___ 9:00–10:15 p.m. (4)
    ___ 10:15 p.m.–12:30 a.m. (3)
    ___ 12:30–1:45 a.m. (2)
    ___ 1:45 a.m.–3:00 a.m. (1)

3. Assuming normal circumstances, how easy do you find getting up in the morning?

    ___ Not at all easy (1)
    ___ Slightly easy (2)
    ___ Fairly easy (3)
    ___ Very easy (4)

4. How alert do you feel after the first half hour after having awakened in the morning?

    ___ Not at all alert (1)
    ___ Slightly alert (2)
    ___ Fairly alert (3)
    ___ Very alert (4)

5. During the first half hour after having awakened in the morning, how tired do you feel?

   ___ Very tired (1)
   ___ Fairly tired (2)
   ___ Slightly tired (3)
   ___ Not at all tired (4)

6. You have decided to engage in some physical exercise. A friend suggests that you do this one hour twice a week, and the best time for him is 7:00 to 8:00 am. Bearing in mind nothing else but your "feeling best" rhythm, how do you think you would perform?

   ___ Would be in good form (4)
   ___ Would be in reasonable form (3)
   ___ Would find it difficult (2)
   ___ Would find it very difficult (1)

7. At what time in the evening do you feel tired and, as a result, in need of sleep?

   ___ 8:00–9:00 p.m. (5)
   ___ 9:00–10:15 p.m. (4)
   ___ 10:15 p.m.–12:30 a.m. (3)
   ___ 12:30–1:45 a.m. (2)
   ___ 1:45 a.m.–3:00 a.m. (1)

8. You wish to be at your peak performance for a test, which you know is going to be mentally exhausting and lasting for two hours. You are entirely free to plan your day, and considering only your own "feeling best" rhythm, which one of the four testing times would you choose?

   ___ 8:00–10:00 a.m. (4)
   ___ 11:00 a.m.–1:00 p.m. (3)
   ___ 3:00–5:00 p.m. (2)
   ___ 7:00-9:00 p.m. (1)

continues

9. One hears about "morning" and "evening" type people. Which one of these types do you consider yourself to be?

    __ Definitely a morning type (4)
    __ More a morning than an evening type (3)
    __ More an evening than a morning type (2)
    __ Definitely an evening type (1)

10. When would you prefer to rise (provided you have a full day's work—8 hours) if you were totally free to arrange your time?

    __ Before 6:30 a.m. (4)
    __ 6:30–7:30 a.m. (3)
    __ 7:30–8:30 a.m. (2)
    __ 8:30 a.m. or later (1)

11. If you always had to rise at 6:00 a.m., what do you think it would be like?

    __ Very difficult and unpleasant (1)
    __ Rather difficult and unpleasant (2)
    __ A little unpleasant but no great problem (3)
    __ Easy and not unpleasant (4)

12. How long a time does it usually take before you "recover your senses" in the morning after rising from a night's sleep?

    __ 0–10 minutes (4)
    __ 11–20 minutes (3)
    __ 21–40 minutes (2)
    __ More than 40 minutes (1)

13. Indicate to what extent you are a morning or an evening active individual.

    __ Very morning active (morning alert and evening tired) (4)
    __ To some extent, morning active (3)
    __ To some extent, evening active (2)
    __ Very evening active (morning tired and evening alert) (1)

chapter eight

IN SICKNESS AND IN HEALTH

M Y FRIEND LISA WAS DIAGNOSED WITH CANCER THREE YEARS AGO. At the time, she was forty-six years old, married, the mother of three children, and an avid athlete. The night before her first major surgery, she and her husband, Pete, came over for dinner. As we were having predinner cocktails, she and I got to talking about sleep (as I said at the beginning of this book, I can't help it!). She told me how in the "pre-kid" phase she and her husband had always snuggled in a double or at most queen-size bed. But (like many of us), once the kids entered the picture, even a queen-size bed didn't feel big enough for them. They had to accommodate the sleeping darlings who might weasel into their beds at some point in the night and in the early morning hours. And as sleep became more and more precious (as is the case for all sleep-deprived parents), the desire for their personal space grew strong—trumping those former desires for closeness and intimacy.

To make matters worse, Lisa is a lifelong insomniac. She comes from a family of similarly sleep-starved sufferers. "I remember as a teenager, I'd wake up in the middle of the night, as I always did, unable to fall back to sleep," she said. "So I'd go to the kitchen and make cookies, just to have something to do. The funny thing is, half the time my dad would be right there with me in the kitchen, since he was also a horrible sleeper."

Like many couples, Lisa and her husband eventually sized up and got a California king bed. Between Lisa's chronic sleeping problems and the kids, it just seemed to make sense. But the solution never sat well with Pete. "I never really wanted a giant bed, because I like to be close at night," he said. "It's like she's sleeping in New Jersey."

Lisa concurred on this point. "In our king-sized bed, I have to roll over at least two full times before I even have the slightest body contact with Pete, but to be honest, most of the time, that was exactly the way I wanted it." It's not that she didn't want intimacy. It's just that the worse her sleep became, and it got progressively worse with the birth of each of their children, Lisa became increasingly protective about her sleep space.

Pete described her sleep habits as downright compulsive. "Oh, I definitely learned to tiptoe around the minefield of Lisa's sleep space and sleep habits. I used to like to stay up later and just unwind by the television and come up to bed after Lisa had fallen asleep. But when her sleep got really bad, she put an end to that, because she'd go ballistic if she had managed to fall asleep and then I came up and woke her up. If I made that mistake, I'd have hell to pay, because she'd end up awake the rest of the night. It used to make me so nervous when she didn't sleep, because I knew the landscape. It was like ten miles of bad road. So she'd be stressed, and I'd get all agitated because I knew that I might get blamed for that too. And touching?" he added. "That was out of the question," for fear that an errant hand brushing against Lisa's skin might awaken her from her chronically light sleep.

This story illustrates just how insomnia can wreak havoc on the shared sleeping experience. Lisa's efforts to protect her sleep, and her stress about not sleeping, were creating tension in her and Pete's relationship. Her fear of its negative effect on her sleep led her to avoid intimacy and physical contact.

But her cancer changed everything. "I just want to be close to him at night," she told me following her multistage treatment involving surgery, chemo, and radiation. It's that need for physical contact that we all desire when we are at our most vulnerable. For Lisa, the nighttime was a time when many of the fears about her diagnosis, the thought of losing her children, her husband, became most intense. And what she needed more than anything was to feel physical connection with her husband. And so did he.

"The first week she got back from the hospital, she just didn't sleep well because she was in a lot of pain and still recovering from surgery," Pete explained. "Now, I didn't sleep that well either, but in a weird way, it brought us closer together. She felt like crap and she was scared, and she just wanted to be held at night. I guess with all that she had been through, she wasn't expecting too much when it came to sleep, so she just needed that comfort. "

Ironically, once the acute surgical pain wore off, Lisa found that despite all the health problems she was still dealing with, she actually was sleeping better. Once she gave up the idea that her sleep environment had to be "perfect" with no disruptions, including human contact, the pressure to sleep (which, as I tell all my insomnia patients, is a death knell for good-quality sleep) wore off. Her need for closeness at night took priority over her concerns about getting enough sleep. And once she gave up that effortful striving for sleep, sleep actually came to her.

Of course Pete, taking on the role of caregiver, saw his own sleep take a hit. His concern for Lisa's health, as well as his need to take on the majority of the responsibility for running the household during Lisa's recovery, all made it harder for him to consistently get a good night's sleep. Pete welcomed that tradeoff, though. He was just happy to have his cuddly wife back in his bed.

As with many couples facing a major health problem, the cancer brought Lisa and Pete's relationship to an entirely different level. It smacked them in the face with the truth of how dependent they are on each other for strength, support, and unconditional love. Nighttime has taken on a whole new meaning, because it's the one time during the day when they can just be together, where they can drop the facade of happy, "everything's going to be okay" faces that they have to present to their children, their friends, and family. They can simply be—be with their fears, be with their sadness, be with the unknowing, and be with each other. It is often when we are in our most vulnerable states, like when we are physically ill or experiencing sadness, loss, or fear, that we most acutely experience a need for closeness at night.

"So will you down-size your bed?" I recently asked Pete.

"No, we'll probably still never get rid of that giant bed because, what the hell? We'd need to get movers! But when we stay at hotels, we always opt for the smaller bed, and we make the effort when sleeping at home to start in the middle, so we are forced to have physical contact. That part is good."

WHEN YOU HURT, I HURT, AND SO DOES OUR SLEEP

Sleep is intricately connected to our physical and mental health. Name an illness, mental or physical, and I can virtually guarantee that sleep disturbance or fatigue is either a symptom of the illness or a side effect of the treatment for whatever ails you. And when you are in a couple and your partner is hurting, be it mental or physical, you also feel the hurt, and both of your sleep can be affected. Thinking about sleep in the context of caregiving provides a window of understanding into our deepest vulnerabilities and the critical role that our partner plays in regulating our sleep, and indeed our health.

I began my work on sleep in couples focusing on healthy, civilian couples, but in the early 2000s, as the wars raged in Iraq and Afghanistan, I couldn't help but watch in awe and empathy as more and more service members returned from war, evidencing both visible and "invisible" wounds of war, including high rates of depression, post-traumatic stress disorder, and suicidality. A commonality across all of these invisible wounds is sleep disturbances. As research was conducted in postdeployed service members, we soon learned that sleep problems were among the most common symptoms reported by military veterans in the aftermath of war. But what about their partners? How was their sleep affected both during and after their partner's return from war, particularly when the partner who returns is different from the one they knew before deployment? My colleagues and I spent five years studying military couples in which one member had served in Afghanistan or Iraq during Operation Enduring Freedom or Operation Iraqi Freedom. What we found was that it wasn't only the service members whose sleep suffered; many partners were exhibiting sleep disturbances as well. In our work, we used the most state-of-the-science, objective measures of sleep and other health outcomes in these couples, but in many ways the most telling information came directly from interviewing both members of the couple and asking about how their sleep had changed during and after deployment.

Jennifer and Mark were a perfect example of the types of stories we heard. Mark was a first sergeant in the army. He had recently returned from his second deployment to Iraq. He and Jennifer had been married for eleven years. They had two children, ages five and two and a half when he returned from his second deployment. When he came home, they were both, of course, ecstatic to be reunited. But as with many military couples, the "honeymoon" period immediately following his return from deployment didn't last for too long. Mark had developed combat-related post-traumatic stress disorder, with severe nightmares being one of the cardinal symptoms of the disorder. As Jennifer described it: "He would just bolt awake in the middle of the night, sometimes yelling at someone or just screaming at the top of his lungs. It scared the hell out of me when it first started happening, because I had no idea what was going on, and you definitely don't expect to be woken up out of sleep by your husband screaming and in a sweat. I wouldn't say I ever got *used* to it, but I guess, once I knew what was happening and we started to have our little routine with me just telling him, 'You're home now. You're safe. I'm here with you,' and so on, it was a little less terrifying for me at least. But I don't think either one of us could really sleep deeply at that point. You just didn't know what might happen in the middle of the night."

For Mark and Jennifer, it was a long battle for Mark to heal from his invisible wounds, through therapy and medication for his PTSD and his sleep problems, but their relationship made it through, and sleep for both of them gradually improved. Regardless of the type of illness a couple is facing, mental or physical, it is critical to recognize the interdependent nature of sleep between the partners, and to recognize that when one partner is ill, the healthy partner, who often assumes the caregiving role, is also highly vulnerable to sleep problems.

THE WORK OF A CAREGIVER IS NEVER DONE

As the population in the US and other developed nations ages, along with advances in medicine, the burden of health care needs has shifted from infectious diseases to chronic diseases. With this shift, there is now increasing recognition that chronic illness is best considered as a shared experience within the context of caregiving relationships. Spouses, partners, and other family members, as opposed to paid medical professionals, are increasingly serving the role of informal caregivers to family members. In fact, national data suggests that sixty-six million Americans serve as informal caregivers for family members, and about two-thirds are women. Substantial research shows that the health and well-being of both the patient and the caregiver are interdependent and bidirectional, and therefore when disease or impairment strikes one partner, it is best viewed and treated at the level of the couple dyad. Not only can a change in the patient's functioning (e.g., increase in pain) affect the caregiver's well-being, but a change in the caregiver's functioning (e.g., worsening sleep quality) can impact the patient's functioning. For example, a sleep-deprived caregiver may forget to give her cognitively impaired husband his medication.

With a growing number of Americans serving as caregivers for a partner, parent, or other loved one with Alzheimer's disease or other cause of dementia, the role of sleep in influencing the health and well-being of both the caregiver and the recipient, as well as the economic and societal burden of the illness, is particularly salient. Nighttime caregiving responsibilities, which can exacerbate caregiver stress, are often the primary reason why families choose to put their loved one in a nursing home or other facility, when otherwise it would be premature to do so. The culprit is often a phenomenon known as "sundowning." This is the common experience when a dementia patient becomes confused and agitated, typically occurring in the late afternoon or evening hours—hence the name. Many have hallucinations that prompt them to want to escape or wander off, which poses a real threat to their safety. As a result, for many caregivers, this becomes the breaking point, prompting the decision to put their loved one into a nursing home or supervised care facility.

For caregivers of all types of illnesses, sleep is often the first thing to go, and the consequences of sleep loss among caregivers can be both immediate (like forgetting to give a medication dose) and more lasting. For example, among the longer-term consequences, research has shown that sleep problems contribute to a poor quality of life, poor physical health outcomes, and depression in caregivers. A summary of the available literature suggests that a whopping 76 percent of caregivers report poor sleep quality, with female caregivers showing even higher rates of poor sleep quality as compared to male caregivers. Caregivers often report that they are constantly physically and mentally exhausted, but still unable to fall asleep. As one caregiver of a dementia patient told me, "It's like I'm always sleeping with one eye open. I might be asleep, but I am still there, right with him. Just waiting to jump up in case he starts wandering again."

There are a number of reasons why caregivers face sleep challenges. A commonly used framework for understanding insomnia is the 3P model, which shows that insomnia develops as a result of the combination of predisposing, precipitating, and perpetuating factors. Let's break each one of these *Ps* down, and I'll give an example that's relevant within the caregiving context.

Predisposing Factors

The first *P* is for predisposing factors, which refers to certain vulnerability factors that render some people more likely to develop sleep problems under certain circumstances, whereas others may not. Unfortunately, the vast majority of caregivers do experience some level of sleep disturbance, but not all do, so it's important to identify some underlying vulnerability factors. Given that most caregivers are women, and that women have higher rates of sleep disturbance than men, gender is a clear predisposing factor that increases the likelihood that women will both serve in a caregiving role and be at greater risk for sleep disturbances.

Similarly, particularly when it comes to dementia caregivers, many are older adults. Increasing age is also associated with greater risk for a number of sleep problems, like trouble falling asleep, changes in sleep timing (with a preference for earlier bedtimes and more early morning awakenings), changes in sleep architecture, and more awakenings during the night, although much of these age-related changes in sleep may be due to declining health more generally.

Other predisposing factors include a family history of insomnia and the presence of other mental or physical health problems in the caregiver. It's important to note that many of the things we consider as predisposing factors are not particularly amenable to change (e.g., try as we might, we can't stop the aging process). In other words, since you can't easily change most of these things, best to focus on other targets that are more amenable to change.

Precipitating Factors

According to the 3P model, among those who are vulnerable (i.e., have at least one predisposing factor), insomnia arises in response to some precipitating event or set of events that causes sleep disruption. For caregivers, the precipitating event or events may include the loved one's initial diagnosis, worsening of symptoms in the loved one, or increasing caregiving responsibilities, particularly if they occur at night. These precipitating events can affect caregiver sleep in a variety of ways. First, the demands and significant stress associated with caregiving activities can take a big toll on sleep. Studies have shown that higher stress levels and the tendency to worry about all the things you have to do can interfere with your ability to fall asleep and sleep well.

A caregiver has to take on a double to-do list, addressing all of his or her own to-dos as well as any to-dos associated with taking care of the loved one, like giving medications at the right time or making it to doctor's appointments. Such never-ending to-dos can make it very difficult to fall into deep, restful sleep. For some, the stress of caregiving can bring with it mood disturbances, including the onset of depression, which itself is associated with sleep disturbances. Sleep problems can also directly lead to depression. Sometimes it's the nighttime caregiving responsibilities themselves and the vigilance that often goes hand in hand that can precipitate sleep problems in the caregiver. Take Ruth and Bill, for example.

The night started out the same as any other night. Ruth and her husband, Bill, went to bed at their usual bedtime of ten p.m., and they both drifted off into slumber. At about one a.m., Bill started to feel some rustling in the bedsheets—enough to wake him up. He turned toward Ruth to discover her in the midst of a convulsion, a symptom of diabetic shock. For loved ones of people with diabetes, this is not an unheard-of scenario, as glucose levels drop during sleep, which can lead to a number of symptoms associated with severe hypoglycemia, including night sweats, nightmares, and, in severe cases like this one, convulsions. In this case, the fact that Ruth and Bill shared a bed meant the difference between life and death. If Bill hadn't been there to recognize the symptoms and to realize the direness of the situation, he very likely might have awoken the next morning to find his wife dead. But after an experience like this, can you imagine how difficult it was for Bill to sleep soundly? Like the soldier who has been trained to be vigilant both day and night, caregivers of all types experience a conditioned vigilance that can make it challenging to sleep at night.

Just like the predisposing factors, many of these precipitating events cannot be changed. Some practical interventions, like hiring a night nurse, if possible and appropriate, might help. But when it comes to treating insomnia, the real intervention is targeted at the third *P*, as these are the things we can change.

Perpetuating Factors

With chronic insomnia, sometimes the initial cause isn't clear, and even if the cause is clear, such as the partner's diagnosis with a severe illness, it is almost irrelevant. That's because the initial cause may have little to do with what is perpetuating the problem and turning insomnia from a transient experience into a chronic and debilitating one. We often have little control over what causes insomnia, but we do have control over what keeps the insomnia going.

This is why I find the treatment of insomnia so rewarding, particularly when it comes to working with clients who are struggling with sleep problems related to caregiving for an ill partner. So much of their life feels out of control. They can't control the diagnosis or course of their partner's illness. They can't control many of the ways their life has been upended as a result of their new role as caregiver. And they can't even control some nighttime disturbances that are directly related to their caregiving responsibilities, like helping their partner walk to the bathroom, administering nighttime medications, or soothing a partner who wakes up from a nightmare because of their post-traumatic stress disorder.

What they can control are the behaviors that they are engaging in. These perpetuating factors are behaviors that are often originally intended to compensate for the problem of sleep loss but can ultimately end up making sleep problems a chronic condition. For example, a caregiver who is feeling burdened and stressed and exhausted all the time as a result of the seemingly boundless responsibilities that keep piling up may try to go to bed earlier or stay in bed later to try to catch up on sleep. They may take naps throughout the day or consume excessive amounts of caffeine or alcohol as strategies to cope with the fact that their sleep is disturbed by their partner's illness. They may start practicing the habit of lying in bed awake at night and running through all of the things that they have to do or didn't get done, or simply use the time to grieve what has been lost since their partner got sick. Sometimes bedtime is the only time when we have the quiet, undisturbed time to let our brains go wild—to think, to plan, to worry, and to feel. Over time, these practices can become habit-forming and can perpetuate the cycle of insomnia.

'TIL DEATH DO US PART

One of the most striking demonstrations of how our relationships regulate our sleep is evidenced during bereavement. As I mentioned in Chapter 3, partners are powerful social zeitgebers ("time keepers"). In turn, the loss of a partner means not only the loss of companionship and love but also the loss of a powerful regulator of our sleep. Scientists studying circadian rhythms have given a name to the profound disruption to the circadian system caused by major social disruptions, including bereavement: *zeitstorer*, meaning "time disrupter." Many bereaved older adults will miss meals and will have erratic bedtimes, in part because those were the things they used to do in tandem with their partner. With the partner gone, they may either forget to engage in these activities or, in some cases, actively avoid engaging in these activities because it reminds them of their late partner. Research further shows that such inconsistency in behavioral patterns, including sleep-wake routines, is a strong predictor of poor mental health outcomes in bereaved adults, including risk for depression.

Dr. Sarah Stahl is a researcher who studies bereavement in older adults and has developed interventions to try to build resilience and protect against poor mental health outcomes in bereaved adults. She has developed an intervention for bereaved older adults that starts simply with choosing a behavior they'd like to improve, like eating healthier or improving their sleep, and taking small steps to achieve those goals. In addition to grieving the loss of the partner, many of the bereaved elders were also facing an identity crisis, as most had been caregivers until the time of the partner's death. So they were facing questions like "Who am I now?" and "What is my purpose?" This loss of identity can add to loneliness and deepen the sense of loss. One of the benefits of monitoring their own health behaviors and setting personal health goals is that it allowed them to reestablish their own sense of identity. This is something we can all learn from when we experience other types of loss, whether it is a loss of a relationship through break-up or death or the loss of another key social role, like a job. Sometimes setting some small personal health goals, like making wake-up time more consistent, can go a long way toward reestablishing that lost sense of self and getting your feet back under you.

One fascinating aspect of Dr. Stahl's work is that while she found a high level of sleep disturbances in the bereaved adults across both genders, she found differences in how bereavement affected men and women's sleep. "Men would tend to wake-up early at four a.m. and think of their spouse and feel sad and not know what to do, so they would just start their day. But for women, it was the act of going to bed that was hardest, since that was when they were more likely to be alone and the bed was a big reminder of their spouse. So they would actively avoid the bedroom, by sleeping on the couch or maybe falling asleep on the couch but then wandering into the bedroom in the middle of the night. Bed was a constant reminder of their loss—even more so than mealtimes. They could skip meals, but they couldn't fully skip sleep because they were so exhausted. The bed and the bedroom forced them to confront the loss, and many just did not feel ready to do that. The bed was just such a powerful reminder of what they lost."

I've seen a similar pattern in my grieving clients. For example, Elizabeth, a seventy-year-old woman, had come to see me about a year after losing her husband, whom she had been married to for forty-three years. Even though she felt that she was "generally getting by okay," she simply could not sleep. "It feels so silly to me," she told me. "I just can't get myself to sleep on my husband's side of the bed. Even if I find myself inching towards the middle, I get sort of antsy and uncomfortable, because it just doesn't feel right to be taking over the space that was for him. Most of the time I just pile up the pillows, so my bed doesn't feel so empty and so I don't roll over too far by accident, then feel bad, and then I definitely won't be able to fall back to sleep." For her, part of the process of working through her grief, and reclaiming some real estate in the bedroom, was to slowly but deliberately donate her husband's clothing to charity, with the help of her son. It took time and also acceptance of the significance of their shared bed and the loss she was experiencing. Ultimately, she learned to find comfort in her bed again.

SHARED SLEEP ACTION PLAN:
Energy Conservation Versus Energy Generation

If you aren't actively caring for a loved one with a serious health problem, you might feel this chapter has been less immediately relevant to you than some of the others, but I'd like to argue that point a bit. First, even in the absence of illness, if you are in a partnership, you are by definition one who gives care. Of course, having a partner with cancer or Alzheimer's disease or a serious mental illness requires a much more intensive level of caregiving than your run-of-the-mill "giving care" to your healthy spouse, but you are already a caregiver, and that role has an impact on your sleep. Second, there is a good chance that some day you will have those more intensive responsibilities associated with what we traditionally think of as caregiving. If you can start practicing some of the skills now, you can see both short-term and long-term benefits. In the words of Rosalynn Carter, "there are only four kinds of people in the world—those who have been caregivers, those who are currently caregivers, those who will be caregivers, and those who will need caregivers." I'd say that pretty much covers all of us.

When it comes to caregiving, one of the biggest things we worry about is caregiver burnout. Caregivers work so hard to make sure their loved ones' needs are met that they can easily neglect their own needs. Over time, that neglect can lead to frustration, exhaustion, anger, illness, and more. For many, while giving care to others comes somewhat naturally, giving care to one's self is a much less natural behavior and one that requires practice. In fact, one of the most important recommendations to avoid caregiver burnout is to practice self-care. That means being kind to oneself and ensuring that you are doing things that are restorative and pleasurable. Self-care isn't just a set of skills for caregivers, though. It's a set of skills for anyone. And the earlier you start building them into your life, the more you'll be able to practice them when you need them most.

There are lots of strategies I'm sure you have heard about for practicing self-care, like getting exercise, getting a massage, taking a yoga class, or doing some other mood-uplifting behavior. For this part of your Shared Sleep Action Plan, I want to offer you a slightly different spin on self-care—one that is derived from a cognitive technique used in insomnia treatment. It's called energy generation, and it can be highly effective at improving mood and energy levels (as the name would suggest). Whether you are caregiving or not, there will be times when you are not sleeping well, so this is a strategy to try to reduce the negative consequences of a bad night of sleep on your daytime functioning. Although this exercise is focused on an individual's behavior, the benefits can extend to both you and your partner, as you both will benefit from having another set of tools in your toolbox to lift your mood and your energy when the going gets tough.

This activity comes from Dr. Allison Harvey, a professor of psychology at the University of California, Berkeley, a dear friend, and one of the most gifted clinicians I know. She has pioneered many of the cognitive techniques used in Cognitive Behavioral Therapy for Insomnia (CBT-I).

Most people believe there is a one-to-one relationship between how much or well you sleep and how much energy you have the next day. Of course, there is some truth to this, as sleep is a major factor contributing to your energy level, not to mention your mood and your health, but it's not the only factor. Sometimes putting too much responsibility for your daily energy on how well you sleep can

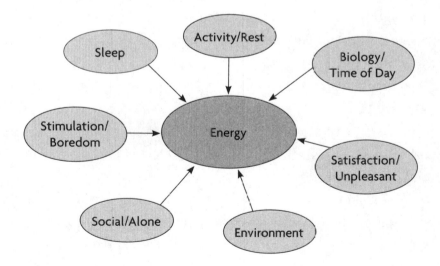

backfire. This is because it puts a lot of pressure on sleep, which can lead to anxiety when you're not getting enough. There are other things that contribute to your energy during the day—your mood, your biology, the environment, how social you are, how stimulated you are, and more.

Having spent my career studying the importance of sleep and spending most of my waking hours extolling the virtues of sleep, I realize the apparent contradiction here in my words, so let me make this crystal clear: I am *not* about to offer you any excuse for sacrificing sleep on a regular basis, as so often happens in our society. Rather, I am saying that it is inevitable that you will face times when life will get in the way of your opportunity to get eight solid hours of sleep on an nightly basis. When this happens, there are things you can do during the daytime that will make the situation worse and increase the chances of having another bad night (as well as a bad day), but there are also things you can do to make it better and a little less painful.

Caregiver burnout is, in large part, the result of chronic and unremitting energy depletion. When everything you do is in the service of those in your care and you spend little focused on those things that fill you, you can suffer. What I try to help my clients with insomnia (caregivers or not) learn to recognize, and what I want to help you learn to recognize, is those things that you do that drain your energy and those things that you do to bring you energy. Of course, sleep is critically important to the energy equation, but it's not everything.

Think about times in your life when you had a miserable night of sleep, but the next day you had something really exciting or important happening, and somehow you woke up and were able to go about your day perfectly fine, with all the energy you needed. How about the night before your wedding perhaps? For many, the night before the big day is far from a restful night of sleep, and yet you'd be hard-pressed to find a bride or groom yawning through the ceremony or napping through the reception (unless perhaps they had a bit too much champagne).

On the flip side, you can probably think of a time when despite getting a good night of sleep, you had to fight to stay awake the next day. Maybe it's when you had to sit through a boring class or a series of Zoom calls, or your day was filled with household chores or completing your tax returns. As much as sleep plays a big role in how much energy we feel during the day, it is also true that what we *do* during the day affects how much energy we feel. Some things we do are energy generators, whereas other things we do are energy drainers. Therefore, the more you stack your day with energy generators, the more likely you are going to feel alert and energized throughout your day, even if you didn't get a great night of sleep the night before.

The problem is that when you hit some bumpy roads in your life—your partner becomes ill, or you hit a rough patch at work—your days often become filled with things you "have to do" (major energy drainers), and you forsake the things you want to do (energy generators). This can create its own sort of vicious cycle, because the more you take this approach, the more likely you are to start cutting back on social activities, exercise, or anything that seems "extra," because you need to hold on to the wee bit of energy you have just to get by. But guess what: in your effort to save energy, your day ends up being filled with all of the boring, mundane, have-to-dos that drain you and is devoid of want-to-dos, which can increase your energy levels. Moreover, our internal biological clocks, which influence our sleep and daytime energy levels, are reinforced by what we do during the day. In turn, the less we do during the day, the weaker the signals to the biological clock, the less alert we feel during the day, and the poorer we sleep at night. The net result is an endless loop of poorly slept nights that don't replenish you and activities during the day that drain you even further.

This exercise is going to help you identify your own energy drainers and energy enhancers. Grab a pen and paper, and make yourself a chart, like the one you see below, with two columns: one for things you do in your day that you genuinely want to do and one for things you do in your day because you have to do them.

Things I Want to Do	Things I Have to Do
Ex. Going for a walk	Ex. Paying bills
Ex. Calling a friend you haven't spoken to for awhile	Ex. Sitting in a boring meeting
Ex. Talking with your partner or coworkers	Ex. Turning down social activities
Ex. Going to the gym	Ex. Skipping exercise

Once you've created your list, it's time to experiment a little over a two-day period. On the first day, spend one three-hour block of time focused on items in the have-to-do list. As you engage in the different activities during each three-hour block, fill out a chart like the one you see below, rating your energy level before and after each activity on a scale of 1–10, with 1 indicating no energy and 10 being supercharged.

DAY 1, BLOCK 1: HAVE-TO-DOS

Strategy	Energy Level Before (0–10)	Energy Level After (0–10)

After those three hours, spend the next three focused on want-to-do items, and conduct the same analysis.

DAY 1, BLOCK 2: WANT-TO-DOS

Strategy	Energy Level Before (0–10)	Energy Level After (0–10)

DAY 2, BLOCK 1: WANT-TO-DOS

Strategy	Energy Level Before (0–10)	Energy Level After (0–10)

Then repeat this entire process for a second day, but this time start with the want-to-dos, and then do the have-to-dos.

After completing the two-day experiment, it's time to look back on your data and reflect. If this experiment worked properly, then you might have noticed more energy boosts from your want-to-dos than your have-to-dos. If that didn't happen, then I'm afraid something went wrong with the experiment (which frankly, happens in science all the time). I am going to sincerely hope that you found a glimmer of evidence that counters the idea that sacrificing your own needs saves you energy so you can serve others. Most of the time, it does not. Most (I'm hoping) will have

DAY 2, BLOCK 2: HAVE-TO-DOS

Strategy	Energy Level Before (0–10)	Energy Level After (0–10)

the aha kind of experience that many of my clients do when they see that on days when they feel really crappy, they often set themselves up for feeling even crappier, because they avoid doing all of the "extra" things, which are by nature all of the "want-to-dos" of life. On the other hand, perhaps you surprised yourself, again as many of my clients have, when they discover that even after nights when they haven't slept well, there are actually things they can do that can make themselves feel better during the day. Generally speaking, it's exactly the opposite of what they would normally do.

Since this is a book about couples and sleep, ideally both you and your partner find an opportunity to run through this experiment yourselves. Then talk about what you discovered. Such discoveries can benefit you both, because there are absolutely going to be times in your coupled existence when one or both of you is feeling sleep-deprived and depleted, so you can support each other by making sure you both have the opportunity to engage in some of the energy-generating want-to-dos—a critical step of self-care and partner care alike.

chapter nine

SNORING AND OTHER
SHARED SLEEP STRUGGLES

CRAIG IS A SUPER ATHLETIC GUY IN HIS MID-FORTIES WHO CAME TO me with severe anxiety, including panic attacks, resulting from the fact that "almost overnight" he stopped being able to sleep.

He and his wife, Jamie, both attended the first session with me. The insomnia first began the night before a big cycling event Craig was competing in. He had been training for months for this event. He had done many similar races in the past, but for the first time in his life, the night before the event, he simply could not fall asleep. As the minutes ticked by throughout the night and this massive physical challenge loomed before him in the morning, his anxiety skyrocketed, making it even harder for him to settle down or have any chance at deep, restful sleep.

"I was right there with him," Jamie described, "and I've never seen him like this before. He just was tossing and turning, and just sounding so frustrated all night long." Craig thinks he probably slept a couple hours that night. When morning came (all too soon), he wanted to just throw the towel in and withdraw from the race, but thanks to Jamie and some of his training buddies who were there with him, they pushed him to do it. And he did.

He didn't set any personal records that day, but he did finish the race. The experience shook him to his core, and it had lasting effects. "It was the first time I felt so totally out of control and I think it just made me super anxious about sleeping and what would happen if I couldn't sleep again," he told me. "I couldn't get rid of the thought that all of a sudden, I could just lose the ability to sleep. Then I just sort of started to panic about how not sleeping would get in the way of everything that I love to do, like competing, going to work, or being a good dad and husband. And sure enough, look where I am now. Since that night, I don't think I've had more than three solid hours of sleep a night for the past six months, and believe me, I've tried everything, from sleeping pills to meditation to having my hormones checked." Jamie nodded in agreement. "It has been tough on all of us, because he just isn't the same guy he was, and I know that kills him."

Chris and Jamie's story (and let's be clear, the story is about both of them) is a common one. Seventy million US adults suffer from poor sleep on a chronic basis, with a diagnosable sleep disorder. Chris's disorder is insomnia, which is by far the most common sleep disorder. But there are all sorts of ways that sleep can go off the rails. According to the *International Classification of Sleep Disorders*, third edition (ICSD-3), the bible of classification and diagnostic criteria for sleep disorders, there are approximately eighty different diagnosable sleep disorders. Broadly speaking, these eighty different sleep disorders span the gamut from not sleeping enough to sleeping too much, sleeping at the wrong time, and a variety of odd or otherwise disruptive behaviors or symptoms that happen during sleep.

This chapter describes the most common sleep disorders—with a focus on how the disorders (and their treatment) affects the sufferer *and* the bed partner. This is important because too often we only focus our efforts and thoughts on the person with the sleep disorder and neglect to consider the impact of the disorder on the partner. Across the spectrum of chronic health conditions from diabetes to cancer to pain, there is increasing recognition that failing to consider the impact of the condition on the partner or failing to integrate the partner into the treatment results in poorer outcomes for both the patient and the partner. This is why more and more interventions in chronic health conditions now incorporate the partner: illness, just like wellness, is embedded in our social context.

Recognizing the social nature of the disorder is all the more critical when it comes to sleep, because unlike other conditions (e.g., pain), in which the symptoms may be experienced sometimes with the partner and sometimes without, when it comes to a sleep disorder, the problematic behavior or symptoms themselves are almost exclusively shared with the partner. Even if the strategy to cope (which many couples do) is to sleep apart, this strategy is not without interpersonal consequences if undertaken in an individualistic rather than couples-focused way. As I've stressed before, there really is no one right or wrong sleeping arrangement for couples, but in the context of sleep disorders, there are definitely some dos and don'ts.

INSOMNIA—TIRED BUT WIRED

Let's start with the big one. Estimates suggest that roughly 10 per-cent of the population experiences chronic insomnia, meaning that the symptoms persist most days of the week for a month or longer. Many of us, however, upward of 30 to 40 percent, will experience insomnia symptoms at one point or another in our lives, but in this case, the symptoms are more transient and don't meet the duration or severity criteria for the diagnosis. Because the experience of in-somnia, at least on a short-term basis, is pretty much ubiquitous for adults, the term "insomnia" is used quite regularly in the vernac-ular to refer to everything related to a bad night of sleep. For that reason, it's important to clarify what insomnia is and what it isn't. Chronic insomnia is a clinical syndrome involving complaints of difficulty falling asleep, difficulty staying asleep, or having poor quality sleep, with associated daytime consequences, like fatigue, mood disturbances, or irritability, and with symptoms lasting for a month or longer.

The first distinction I want to make about insomnia, because it is so often misunderstood, is that the diagnosis is based on the subjective complaint of sleep, not some objective measurement. Far too frequently, I hear people say, "I really need a sleep study, because I have insomnia," or "My wife needs a sleep study because she doesn't sleep at all." Truth is, sleep studies, otherwise known as overnight polysomnography (or PSG), are not routinely recom-mended or, in most cases, necessary for diagnosing insomnia. A sleep study typically involves coming into a laboratory (although it can also be done at home in some cases) and getting wired up with electrodes and other measures to record your brain waves, the oxygen level in your blood, your heart rate and breathing, as well as eye and leg movements while you sleep. No part of this assessment is necessary for the diagnosis of insomnia, except when it helps to rule out other suspected sleep disorders, like obstructive sleep apnea (OSA), which I'll discuss below.

While we are on the topic, here is another interesting tidbit about sleep studies. Often when people hear what a sleep study entails—going into a laboratory or clinic, getting hooked up to a bunch of electrodes while some technician monitors you throughout the night, and trying to sleep in a completely unfamiliar environment—they think, "There is no way I am going to sleep at all!" While some people do struggle to sleep during their sleep study, when some people with insomnia have a sleep study done (despite it not being recommended except as a rule-out for other sleep disorders), to their utter shock and disbelief they sometimes sleep *better* than they do at home. This has been referred to as paradoxical insomnia or sleep-state misperception, meaning that despite the individual's report of having severely compromised sleep quality, the objective measure of sleep fails to document significant issues with difficulty falling asleep, difficulty staying asleep, or having poor sleep quality.

Let me just say, as a clinician, I have always cringed at the concept of paradoxical insomnia because it can unfortunately be used to imply that the individual's experience of poor sleep quality somehow matters less than what the objective measures show or, worse yet, that they are simply complainers. Talk about invalidating. I bring this up as a cautionary tale to all partners of people with insomnia. I implore you, for the good of your relationship, do *not* tell your partner who is complaining of not being able to sleep or of having poor, unrefreshing sleep, "Well, when I woke up in the middle of last night, you were fast asleep." This is not helpful, and it's a surefire way to get your partner feeling invalidated, judged, and defensive.

Not only is it incorrect to assume that just because there is a discrepancy between objective and subjective measures of sleep, the objective measure is necessarily the superior or more accurate measure, but it's also entirely possible that one of the reasons why some people with insomnia actually sleep better in the laboratory than at home is due to the fact that the new environment, albeit a lab, doesn't have all of the negative, learned associations with bad sleep that one's home environment has. More on that below, but now I want to talk about how I tend to treat people with insomnia, because if you or your partner suffers from it, there are some strategies based on this treatment you can try on your own that might help. For persistent or severe insomnia, however, I do recommend seeking professional help from a clinician with behavioral sleep medicine training.

COGNITIVE BEHAVIORAL THERAPY FOR INSOMNIA (CBT-I)

Clients who come to me are looking for behavioral (nonmedication) treatment for insomnia, specifically a type of treatment known as Cognitive Behavioral Therapy for Insomnia, or CBT-I. Often they come to me because they have a specific preference to avoid medication treatment, or more often because they have already tried a litany of prescribed or unprescribed sleep aids, all of which have failed. The good news, in either case, is that CBT-I has been found in study after study to be as effective and more enduring than any medication out there for insomnia, and without the side effects. The treatment involves changing thoughts and behaviors about sleep that perpetuate the insomnia problem. Thoughts and worries about how the insomnia is going to negatively affect your life are understandable, but unfortunately only serve to ramp up anxiety, which makes sleep even more difficult.

CHANGING OUR FOCUS—STOP TALKING ABOUT IT SOOOOO MUCH

I often talk to my clients about the "insomnia brain," which is hyper-focused on sleep, making their insomnia truly not just a sleep problem but a twenty-four-hour-a-day problem. From the time they wake up to the time they fall asleep, the only thought for my struggling clients is "Will I ever fall asleep? And what will happen if I don't?" And often, supportive partners are right there with them, not just along for the ride but active participants in the hyper-focus on insomnia.

Craig, for example, had constant, intrusive thoughts like, "I can't function if I don't sleep. I won't be able to do all of the things I love to do anymore." In our work together, we had to challenge those beliefs by setting up behavioral experiments to find out if those beliefs were true. Of course, there is some truth to such negative thoughts, because we all know that not sleeping well makes you feel pretty crummy. But does feeling crummy equate to Craig's thought that he *can't function*? I had him test that belief out in his daily life, so he could start identifying examples of when he slept really poorly but somehow managed anyway. Even in terms of the race itself, on the day following the onset of his insomnia, he may not have set a personal best time, but he showed up. He finished the race. That contradicts the idea that "I can't function," which—let's face it—is a catastrophic belief but common when a person struggles with insomnia.

Given that insomnia is at least, in part, a thought disorder, in that chronic, ruminative, worrisome thoughts about insomnia can exacerbate the sleeping problem and make it more lasting, partners also play a role in how much the person's sleeping problem becomes the focus of their daily lives. Partners—as well as coworkers, family members, and others—will repeatedly and frequently check in with the individual with insomnia: "How did you sleep last night? How is your insomnia?" They'll offer up suggestions for the latest and greatest treatment options that they heard on the news or from their dear Aunt Sally or whomever. This is a perfectly natural and humane thing to do—we are trained as kind and thoughtful human beings to express our care and concern for our loved ones, by checking in on the thing that ails them and trying to offer strategies to help. The problem is that this constant focus on insomnia, which is already part of the problem happening internally in the mind of the insomnia patient, only gets worse when it also becomes the primary or regular topic of conversation in the external world.

This was a real aha moment for Jamie and Craig when I brought it up to them. Their pattern over the previous six months had been for Jamie to start each day by asking Craig, "How did you sleep last night?" Inevitably, he would tell her yet again that it was miserable and how he didn't know how he would make it through the day. This cycle of negativity started each morning, and it literally set the tone for the day—for both of them. In his office, as well, Craig's colleagues would inquire about his sleep, telling him about their own sleep struggles and whatever newfangled treatment they found to treat their sleep problems. Although well-intentioned, this persistent focus on Craig's sleep problem served to magnify the presence and significance of his insomnia, making the consequences feel even more dire and further exacerbating Craig's anxiety about sleep.

I encouraged Craig and Jamie to begin with a moratorium on questions about his sleep for just a one-week period, and I encouraged Craig to track his anxiety levels on a daily basis. Both admitted that at first, it felt "really weird." "I seriously had to hold myself back from saying anything in the mornings," said Jamie. "And at first, I felt like I was being so insensitive. But then it kind of occurred to me that I honestly didn't need to ask to know if it was a 'bad night' or a 'good night' for him. It was kind of obvious. But at the same time, it was kind of nice to not start everyday with the rundown of how miserably he slept." Craig, too, acknowledged that "we kind of had this habit together of starting the day on such a downer. Even though I really wanted Jamie to ask me how I was doing, the experiment taught me that I wasn't really getting any benefit from her asking me the same thing every day and me responding with the same depressing stuff every day."

The key here for both of them was that they made the contract together to have the moratorium on questions about his sleep. This way it was clear that Jamie's behavior change of not asking about his insomnia was not a reflection of not caring or not validating his experience, and Craig's not talking about his sleep was not a reflection of him holding back from her. Rather, these behavior changes reflected a mutually agreed upon decision to experiment with a new behavior, recognizing that their former pattern was clearly not helping the situation. My favorite line in therapy—and in my own life—when considering whether to change or continue a given behavior is, "How well is this behavior working for you?" We often have lots of reasons for maintaining the status quo: it feels like the natural thing to do, and there is comfort in that. But simply asking,

"How well is this working?" can be helpful in getting us unstuck from behaviors that don't serve any real purpose—or at least a good purpose.

SLEEP RESTRICTION—COUNTERINTUITIVE YET EFFECTIVE

When people start sleeping poorly, they also frequently start engaging in behaviors that are intended to fix or cope with the problem, and partners are often right there beside them, supporting such behaviors. Paradoxically, these behaviors, like spending more time in bed, or reducing activities during the day, end up making the insomnia worse. Some of the most well-intentioned and supportive partners, like Jamie, may inadvertently perpetuate the problem by encouraging her partner with insomnia to "sleep in" or "go to bed early" to try to catch up on sleep. In our first session, Craig acknowledged Jamie for how supportive she has been throughout this ordeal, saying, "Jamie is amazing. She knows when I am really suffering with this and will just let me stay in bed, and she'll deal with the kids in the morning. And we have had to cancel so many social plans with friends, because as much as she may want to go, she knows I just can't handle it right now."

My job as the therapist in this case is kind of tricky, because I have to acknowledge that while of course what Jamie is doing comes from a place of support and love for her husband, unfortunately it simply isn't helping. It could be making the situation worse. Intuitively, it makes sense that if you are sleeping poorly, then the first thing you should do is spend more time in bed, right? In other words, increase the window of opportunity for sleep, so at least you can catch some sleep within that window. It turns out this is exactly what *not* to do when it comes to insomnia.

	Insomnia	Sleep Deprivation
Sleep Opportunity	👍	👎
Sleep Ability	👎	👍

In fact, a key but often overlooked criterion of insomnia is that the sleep problems exist despite an adequate opportunity for sleep. This is an important distinction between insomnia and an increasingly prevalent but qualitatively different sleep disorder, called behaviorally induced insufficient sleep syndrome (BISS). The latter (BISS) refers to the common practice in our 24/7 society to restrict our opportunity for sleep—because of long work hours or shift work schedules or simply by choice—in favor of other activities, like watching TV or scrolling through social media. The difference here, which is critical because it directly relates to the treatment of insomnia versus BISS, is that in insomnia, the opportunity for sleep is adequate, but the ability to sleep is impaired. In contrast, in BISS, the ability to sleep is intact, but the opportunity is restricted.

Therefore, one of the most powerful behavioral strategies for reducing insomnia, especially when used in conjunction with other CBT-I techniques, is to restrict time in bed, so the time you spend in bed more closely matches the time you are actually sleeping. In BISS, it's all about removing the barriers to sleep opportunity and taking even small steps to extend the sleep period. In either case, partners can play an important role. Sometimes, what comes most naturally, like telling your partner with insomnia to spend more time in bed, might be exactly what the doctor *didn't* order.

When it comes to insomnia, I tell partners like Jamie that the best way to support their partner is to encourage them to stick with their prescribed sleep schedule (set by me, the clinician) and encourage them to stay active and engaged in their life, even on the days when they have slept the worse. This also teaches their brain that they're not going to let insomnia overtake their life. The more they avoid doing the things that give them pleasure or enjoyment or a sense of having accomplished something, the more they give the insomnia a power over them that can feel overwhelming and debilitating, and will most certainly make the problem worse.

As simple as this strategy sounds, sleep restriction does have side effects associated with it—namely, daytime sleepiness. So it should not be undertaken lightly, as it could be contraindicated for some people, like those with bipolar disorder or mania—sleep restriction can make it worse—or those operating heavy machinery, for whom excessive sleepiness could be deadly. Ideally, sleep restriction should happen as part of a comprehensive behavioral treatment strategy, guided by a trained professional.

STIMULUS CONTROL—RESERVING YOUR BEDROOM FOR TWO THINGS AND TWO THINGS ONLY

We learn behaviors based on associations between a stimulus or set of stimuli, like a bedroom, and a certain response—in this case, sleep, or lack thereof. If you ever took an introductory psychology course, you probably heard about this concept while learning about Pavlov's dog. Pavlov conducted an experiment in which he would always ring a bell when he fed his dog. Eventually, the bell alone, even without the presence of food, would be enough to get the dog to salivate. Pavlov's dog had "learned" that the bell meant food. In the same vein, a person with insomnia *learns* that all of the usual cues in the bedroom environment are signals for yet another bad night of sleep. So when that person goes into a totally unfamiliar environment, even a lab, it is possible that they could actually sleep better, because those usual cues for bad sleep are no longer present.

From a treatment perspective, stimulus control can be a powerful way to reduce insomnia, sometimes involving changing the environment. I don't mean a full remodel of the bedroom is necessary, but maybe even just changing the comforter, reducing clutter, or some other decorative aspect of the room might help. Even more importantly, stimulus control is about changing behaviors that happen in bed. The goal is to keep the bed and bedroom for sleep and sex only, so that the brain can develop a strong, learned association between the bed and sleep or sex. When you lie in bed wishing you were asleep, scrolling through Facebook, watching TV, or staring at the ceiling in frustration, as so many people with insomnia do, you weaken the association for the brain. With a weak association comes a weak behavior, and it sets the stage for feeling frustrated and anxious—which is antithetical to sleep. Given that this technique involves restricting activities in bed to sleep and sex, both of which presumably involve the partner, having the partner onboard with this strategy is critical but too often neglected.

In Craig's case, he was spending upwards of nine hours in bed, but only sleeping about six hours, at most, per night. A key outcome that we focus on in the sleep world is "sleep efficiency," which is simply the time spent actually asleep divided by the time in bed, expressed as a percentage (i.e., × 100). So Craig's sleep efficiency, on average, was 67 percent. In other words, his sleep grade would be a D. He was failing. Most of us don't like to fail at whatever we set our minds to, whether it be a class or sleep. When we fail, we feel frustrated, angry, upset, or anxious. I explained this to Craig and asked, "So what are you doing for those three hours in bed that you are trying to sleep but failing?" He thought about it and said, "Not much really. Just mostly lying there, trying to get myself to fall back to sleep, or sometimes I might start thinking about work or whatever I had to do the next day." Bingo. This is exactly why it does not work to spend more time in bed when you have insomnia. All those hours of lying there wishing he was asleep, and getting increasingly anxious and frustrated, was sending the message to his brain that the bed was a place to worry, feel frustrated or anxious, or simply be awake. Hardly the strong learned association we are aiming for between the bed and sleep. And when you think about how busy our waking lives are, the last thing we want to teach our brain is: "Just wait until bedtime, when you have eight wide open hours, with little to no distractions, to do nothing but think and worry!" You can imagine how quickly a harmful habit like that can take hold, when you are spending lots of time in bed and sleeping only a fraction of it.

The technique of stimulus control goes something like this: If you are awake in bed for a half an hour or longer (use your best guess, and *don't* look at the clock—nothing ever good comes out of finding out what time it is if you are awake in the middle of the night), get out of bed and do something ideally in another room that is distracting but relaxing and can be done in relatively low-light conditions (like with a lamp). I generally tell my clients to avoid TV watching, since there is a lot of light exposure from TVs, but if that is a last resort, I'd rather they be doing that than continuing to lie in bed awake. The key is to engage in the behavior until you actually become sleepy again. At that point, you can return to bed and see if you are ready to fall back to sleep. If you return to bed and are unable to fall back to sleep, repeat the process. It is by no means an easy technique to follow. I mean, who really wants to get out of their cozy bed at three in the morning, or whenever it may be, and go read a book or anything else for that matter? I get it, and I always remind my clients that they will probably curse me as they practice this technique, but it happens to work when followed consistently.

For Craig, we developed a plan for him to have a number of different middle-of-the-night activities at the ready, including a book, a crossword puzzle, the sports section of the newspaper, and a few magazines, so that he could experiment and have a number of options to choose from. Jamie, being the supportive wife that she is, asked how she could be involved. In the past, when Craig would wake up in the middle of the night and get frustrated, he would often wake her up so she would talk to him or give him a massage or even have sex, in hopes that it would settle him down and help him to sleep. It didn't work, and Jamie had never wanted to sign up for that kind of middle-of-the-night martyrdom. We talked this through together, again acknowledging that Jamie was doing everything she could to be supportive but that codependent behavior wasn't working. Educating Jamie as well about the value of stimulus control and that it was something Craig was going to have to do on his own, though she could support him, was an important step in getting them both aligned to change these habits they had formed as a couple. And ultimately it helped Craig sleep better.

As Craig progressed through treatment and he and Jamie both learned to break the habits that were perpetuating the insomnia, and at the same time learned new habits to overcome the insomnia, they both felt empowered and more connected. And I'm happy to report that Craig has raised his sleep grade from a D to most nights being A's since our initial work together.

OBSTRUCTIVE SLEEP APNEA—LOUD SNORES AND SHARP ELBOWS

Although insomnia is the most common sleep disorder, obstructive sleep apnea (OSA, or referred to simply as apnea) and its most common symptom, snoring, probably gets the most attention when it comes to couples' sleeping challenges. We've all heard the stories and know examples from friends and families, if not in our own bedrooms, about how OSA and snoring are the banes of many couples' existence and likely contributors to many relationships' demise. If you've ever shared a bed with a snorer, you know how painful it is.

Thankfully, my husband is not a snorer. But as a child, I shared a room with my grandfather during a trip, and for the first time I was exposed to what I now suspect was severe sleep apnea. For my nine-year-old self, it was terrifying. To be fast asleep and suddenly awakened with the loudest, most noxious snore, followed by a gasp for air, coming from my grandfather sleeping in the other bed in the hotel room—it didn't sound human! It was so jarring that it made my heart beat faster, which itself would have made it hard for me to fall back to sleep. Of course, that was the least of my problems, because it wasn't just a one-time jolt: once my grandfather's snoring got started, it became an all-night affair. I think it was the first time in my young life that I experienced significant sleep deprivation, and it lasted for the entire trip.

This scenario plays out in roughly twenty-five million bedrooms in the US per night. At least, that's how many people are diagnosed with OSA. It's likely that a lot more sufferers are out there keeping their partner awake without an actual diagnosis, because like most sleep disorders, OSA remains woefully underdiagnosed.

OSA and its primary symptom of loud snoring or gasping or choking for air at night are the butt of many jokes and the bane of many bed partners' existence, but left untreated, OSA is a serious health problem linked to hypertension, cognitive decline, heart disease, and stroke. And as any bedpartner of a snorer will tell you, the patient with OSA isn't the only one who suffers. OSA has been called a "disease of listeners" in recognition of the fact that bed partners are often the hidden casualties of the disorder. They experience the profound consequences of a secondhand sleep disorder, including disrupted sleep, poorer quality of life, increased pain symptoms, depression, and poorer relationship quality. Women sleeping with snorers are three times more likely to have insomnia as compared to women sleeping with nonsnorers. Studies further suggest that if you sleep with a snorer, you can blame your partner for up to 50 percent of your sleep disruptions, and it may even contribute to hearing loss.

For couples coping with apnea, the shared sleep struggles can become the focal point of frustration, anger, and, for some, downright aggression. The bed partner, starved for a decent night of sleep because they are nightly being robbed by the snoring spouse, often feels anger and resentment, and they may opt to forsake the bedroom altogether just to get a few decent winks of shut-eye. Often, the offending partner, either out of shame or defensiveness, will make a joke of the situation or will otherwise try to downplay the impact on their bedpartner. In turn, this can make the partner feel invalidated. A friend of mine, a sleep researcher himself, says he attributes the demise of his relationship in large part to his partner's snoring.

"Actually, it wasn't the snoring itself, although that was horrible. But it was that he wouldn't take it *or me* seriously, even when I told him I felt like I was being tortured every night by being awakened by his snoring every time I fell back to sleep. He just kind of blew it off or made some sort of joke about it. And at the end of the day, I just had it. It's one thing for him not to care about his own health, but he literally just blew off the fact that this was also making me miserable. It became bigger than just the sleep that was missing. It was a sign to me that he really didn't give a damn about my feelings." This is a common theme among couples dealing with apnea, and why I strongly encourage couples to deal with this issue head-on, lest a cycle of invalidation, resentment, and withdrawal ensues.

Of course, the most obvious sign of withdrawal and a frequent coping strategy of many bed partners sleeping with snorers is to vacate the bedroom. Estimates suggest that anywhere between 25 and 40 percent of couples opt to sleep apart; snoring in one or both partners is the primary culprit responsible for solo sleeping arrangements among couples. As I've said throughout this book, there is no one prescription for sleeping arrangements for all couples, and while there is nothing inherently wrong with choosing to sleep apart if that helps you and your partner sleep better, it's all in how it's done.

Far too many couples arrive at the decision to sleep apart without actually *making* a decision about it. There's little to no conversation about it and no dialogue about how this might affect their intimacy. It just becomes an act of desperation, with one partner angrily stomping out of the room and to the couch, in hopes to get some shut-eye. Under such circumstances, the other partner may be left feeling hurt and rejected, and intimacy for the couple may suffer.

Despite the fact that snoring is known to disrupt the bed partner's sleep quality, the limited research that has looked at whether sleeping apart actually improves the bed partner's sleep suggests that it doesn't really work. In one study female partners of snorers slept one night with their partner and one night alone in their home environments, and researchers measured their sleep on both nights. To the surprise of many (including the women who participated in the study, I suspect), there was little improvement in their sleep on the night when they slept apart from their partner.

Several years ago, I had the opportunity to do an ABC Nightly News special in which I went into the home of ABC's medical correspondent, Dr. Jennifer Ashton, in order to investigate the impact of her husband's snoring on her sleep, as she firmly believed that his snoring was the culprit of her insomnia. We brought in a sleep tech I had worked with in Pittsburgh, and he hooked them both up with an in-home polysomnography study so we could measure all the things we normally would in a lab, but this time in their usual bedroom environment. On one night, Jennifer shared a bed with her husband, and on the next night she slept alone. My job was to review and interpret their sleep studies and share the results with them (and the TV audience) on camera. The results were striking, particularly to Jennifer. On the night she slept with her husband, she did wake up quite a few times, but it was honestly not much different from the number of times she woke up on her own. In other words, her insomnia was her own. It was revealing for both of them, because his snoring had in many ways become this focal point of frustration and resentment, and although it was contributing to some of her sleep loss, it wasn't the only factor to blame. Nevertheless, for many couples, the stress, tension, and conflict caused by OSA and snoring can put the relationship in jeopardy.

There is good news: treatment for OSA works. Successful treatment of apnea can benefit the patient's sleep and overall health and functioning as well as the patient's bed partner. Studies have shown that, after successful treatment for sleep-disordered breathing, both partners' sleep improves, their relationship satisfaction improves, and so does their intimacy.

I should note that this is a treatment that only works when you use it. Herein lies the problem. Fifty percent of individuals prescribed continuous positive airway pressure (CPAP) treatment, which is the front-line treatment for OSA, stop using the treatment within a week of getting started, and up to 80 percent of individuals are nonadherent over time. I'll be honest, CPAP treatment, which involves wearing a mask-like device that forces air into the person's airways to keep them open and reduces the breathing problems associated with OSA, is not pretty, sexy, or convenient. But both partners' being sleep-deprived is also not pretty, sexy, or convenient.

And let's be honest: for most couples, sex is most likely to occur before they go to sleep, so if you have apnea, there's absolutely no reason not to put your sexiest (and well-rested self) forward at the beginning of the night, have sex, then put on your mask to ensure that both you and your partner get a good night's sleep. You can then wake up the next day feeling refreshed, awake, and better equipped to be the best partner you can be.

CPAP isn't for everyone, but there is also good news here. Other treatments exist, including oral appliances that help to shift the jaw forward as well as surgeries to remove some of the extra skin in the upper palate of the mouth, which often contributes to apnea and other problems of sleep-disordered breathing. These are good options for some people. For others, dropping excess body weight through healthy diet and exercise can also make a difference, as the wider our waistbands grow, the more prone we are to sleep-disordered breathing at night.

Whatever strategy you use to overcome the snoring or sleep-disordered breathing problem, the key is to approach this as a "we" problem. Couples who are able to discuss how snoring affects both of them in an open and honest but nonjudgmental way are better able to problem solve and to keep focused on what truly matters—the health and well-being of both partners and the health of the relationship. Spouses can be supportive and encourage the partner to stick with treatment, even when it is not particularly pleasant.

My colleague Dr. Kelly Baron, of the University of Utah, conducted a study that demonstrated this very point. She found that positive partner support, including doing things like helping the partner with apnea to clean the CPAP machine or providing encouraging (not nagging) comments, was associated with more use of the machine. Relationship conflict was associated with lesser use. You can see how this might play out. The more the person with apnea feels picked on, nagged on, or otherwise harangued, the more they may choose to just say, "Screw it," because after all, it is not a particularly easy treatment to stick with. None of us like to be criticized when we feel we are doing our best. In contrast, if you have a partner saying, "How do we manage this problem together?," it's much less blame-oriented, much more supportive, and much more likely to encourage collaboration and success at achieving the desired behavior. Dr. Baron and I are in the process of developing a treatment for couples in which one partner has OSA. The treatment is called We-PAP to reflect the "we"-centered approach that can help couples reframe this challenge to be a shared experience, with both shared challenges and shared goals. We know from many other chronic health conditions, like pain and even cancer, that addressing these issues that affect both partners can result in better treatment outcomes and better relationship health, as well as better overall health of the couple.

Now that I've covered the two primary sleep disorders (insomnia and OSA) that have been researched the most extensively, though still limitedly in the context of couples, I will briefly touch on some of the other major categories of sleep disorders and how the partner can be affected. This is not intended to be an exhaustive discussion of any of these sleep disorders, because I could fill a book with that, but the goal is to raise awareness of how disordered sleep in its many forms can have a powerful impact on the partner and the relationship functioning of the couple.

NARCOLEPSY

As I mentioned earlier, sleep disorders can broadly be characterized into problems of sleeping too little, sleeping too much, sleeping at the wrong time, and other nocturnal behaviors or symptoms that disrupt sleep. When it comes to sleeping too much, narcolepsy is a key example.

Narcolepsy is thought of as a "true" disorder of sleep, in that sleep intrudes into waking behavior. The person with narcolepsy feels excessively sleepy most of the time and also has sudden attacks of sleep, regardless of what they may be doing. In its classic form, narcolepsy is also associated with a symptom called cataplexy, which is a temporary (lasting up to several minutes), uncontrollable loss of muscle tone (i.e., paralysis). Cataplexy is usually triggered by intense emotions, usually positive ones such as laughter or excitement, but also fear, surprise, or anger.

Narcolepsy is a relatively uncommon disorder, affecting 135,000 to 200,000 people in the US, but as with many sleep disorders, it often goes undiagnosed. Because I did my clinical training at the sleep medicine center at the University of Pittsburgh, which is widely known and one of the oldest clinical and research centers focused on sleep, I had the opportunity to evaluate several patients either newly diagnosed or receiving ongoing treatment for narcolepsy.

Nathan was a patient I saw many years ago. His story has stuck with me, mostly because he was such a pleasant and easygoing guy and a great storyteller. He told me about how, when he was a teenager and long before he was diagnosed, he had his first experience of cataplexy as a competitive swimmer. Recall that cataplexy involves temporary paralysis and is triggered by strong emotions, like anxiety or fear. Now picture him standing on the swim block ready to dive in, and the official shoots off a gun to start the race. As he describes it, his legs just gave out beneath him, and he fell into the water like a bag of cement. "Luckily it didn't last too long, because I don't think anyone would have saved me, because they just thought I was messing around."

Nathan's sense of humor made it easy to make light of some of these clearly disruptive if not potentially life-threatening situations, but he also admitted how severely his symptoms affected his family life as he entered adulthood. "Just think about all of the major events in life. The good ones. Like getting married or seeing your baby for the first time, or laughing with your wife. I never know if I'm going to conk out for a second. It makes you always have to have your guard up some, and it sure makes it hard to really let yourself experience those kinds of emotions, but sometimes it's unavoidable. I'm seriously lucky. I have an amazing wife who at this point is more of an expert on narcolepsy than most doctors out there. So she understands that, if I doze off while we are in the middle of a conversation, to not take it personally. But it took us a long time to get there."

Not surprisingly, individuals with narcolepsy face a number of interpersonal and economic challenges, including relationship problems and unemployment. It is critical for partners, like Nathan's wife, and other family members to become educated on the disorder so that they can distinguish the symptoms (e.g., falling asleep at an inopportune time) from a personal affront.

RESTLESS LEGS SYNDROME

When we think of sleep, we think of it as a peaceful and quiet resting state. But for some people and their partners with whom they share a bed, it can be anything but restful. Take restless legs syndrome (RLS), for example. RLS is a neurological disorder, affecting anywhere between 4 and 14 percent of the population, though this wide range in estimates is a clear indicator of how underdiagnosed and inconsistently diagnosed the disorder is. Regardless of where the true prevalence lies, these numbers belie the many more sufferers who are the bed partners of those with RLS. Their sleep suffers too.

The primary symptom of RLS is a tingling, "creepy-crawly," or otherwise uncomfortable sensation in the legs, with an urge to move to relieve the discomfort. It can be a nightly agony for both partners, as the discomfort or twitchiness begins right at bedtime and is only relieved when the individual gets up and out of bed, then promptly returns when they go back to bed. This can make bedtime for both partners a state of constant motion rather than a place of rest. A recent study of RLS patients and partners' experiences found that 20 percent of partners reported that the RLS negatively affected their relationship, and 85 percent of patients and 33 percent of partners reported that disrupted sleep was where they experienced the biggest impact of the disorder.

PARASOMNIAS AND REM BEHAVIOR DISORDER

At a further extreme are other types of sleep disorders, including parasomnias, which include a wide variety of behaviors that happen during sleep, and rapid eye movement (REM) behavior disorder (RBD), in which people physically act out their dreams. In both cases, the sleep disorder not only threatens the sleep of the bed partner but can also threaten their physical health and safety. The major difference between parasomnias and RBD is that parasomnias typically occur in non–rapid eye movement (NREM) sleep stages, whereas RBD, as the name suggests, occurs during REM sleep. The fascinating—and frightening—aspect of RBD is that during normal REM sleep, which is the type of sleep in which our most vivid dreams occur, we experience temporary muscle atonia, otherwise known as paralysis. This is quite handy because the muscle atonia is what keeps us from acting out the bizarre and sometimes dangerous behaviors in our dreams. But in RBD, muscle atonia doesn't happen, so the person enacts their dreams, including violent ones. The good and the bad news is that RBD is very rare (less than 1 percent of the general population) and generally associated with a neurodegenerative disease, like Parkinson's or certain types of dementia.

In my practice, I have mostly seen cases of parasomnias, in a variety of shapes and sizes, from sleepwalking or talking—including having full dialogues with a partner, despite the fact that the sleeptalker is completely unaware or not conscious of the dialogue—to sleep eating, as well as more violent behaviors like thrashing, kicking, or punching.

Among the veterans I have worked with who have returned from war with PTSD, scenes from the battlefield often replay in their nightmares, much to the terror of their bed partners. For example, Mark and Jennifer, whom I introduced in Chapter 6, had to make some tough decisions for a time to protect Jennifer's safety at night. Mark's nightmares often caused him to violently kick his legs or thrash his arms about. "One time during one of his nightmares," Jennifer said, "he just sort of threw his arm out which was balled up in a fist and it got me directly in the jaw. You have no idea what that is like to be fast asleep and get a fist to the jaw. And it's coming from your loving husband. The worst part was when he came to. He just couldn't believe he hurt me. He would never hurt me if he were awake." This was a real wake-up call for both of them. "To be honest," Mark admitted, "if you knew what some of my nightmares looked like, the scariest thing to me was thinking about what else I might have done."

Addressing the partner's safety concerns is the first precaution that couples dealing with parasomnias or RBD need to take. In Jennifer and Mark's case, it meant sleeping apart for a time, which was challenging for both of them but necessary, as Mark worked through his PTSD treatment. "As much as I needed her at night, I just knew I couldn't stand the guilt of hurting her again, so we decided this was what we had to do during that time," Mark said. Some couples take other steps, like putting a chime or bell on the door, in case the individual has a tendency to roam during sleepwalking episodes, potentially causing themselves harm.

This chapter is a bit of a whirlwind tour of the major types of sleep disorders and the effects on the bed partner as well as the patient. Although this is by no means an exhaustive description of all the ways sleep can go awry, it should provide a hint as to the complexity of sleep and how partners are often unwitting casualties during the third of their lives they share a bed. It's also a wake-up call that medical providers need to do a better job of diagnosing and treating sleep disorders, as they remain woefully underdiagnosed, and the consequences of untreated sleep disorders are vastly underestimated, especially when we fail to take into account the impact on the bed partners. Rather than making light of or jokes about the nuisance or snoring or other partner-caused sleep disturbances, it's time to take these issues seriously, and first and foremost determine if there is an underlying sleep disorder.

SHARED SLEEP ACTION PLAN:
Coping with Your or Your Partner's Sleep Disorder

If you suspect you or your partner has a sleep disorder, I strongly suggest you discuss it with a doctor or seek evaluation at a sleep medicine clinic to determine if you have a diagnosable condition. In the meantime, for this part of the Shared Sleep Action Plan, I offer you some general strategies followed by some practical tips for bed partners whose sleep may be suffering from the noise, movements, or other disturbances.

General Strategies

1. If your bed partner's snoring, gasping, movements, or restless sleep is keeping you up most nights of the week, and it has been going on for a month or longer, let that be a strong signal to encourage your partner to see their medical

provider to determine if they have a sleep disorder and get treatment if necessary.

2. If they are diagnosed with a sleep disorder, you can go a long way to support them by treating the disorder as a "we" problem rather than a "you" problem. In other words, think of ways to problem solve together and offer encouragement as opposed to nagging. Be collaborative in your approach to dealing with the sleep disorder, so it feels as if you are in this as a team.

3. Try not to make your relationship revolve around the sleep disorder. Have fun and do enjoyable things together, and, if necessary, schedule a moratorium on talking about the sleep disorder or problems it has caused.

Practical Tips

1. Invest in the best mattress you can afford. Bigger is better if movement issues are disrupting your sleep. The key to a good mattress, if your partner's movements or restlessness is keeping you up, is to find a mattress that minimizes displacement, or the transmission of one partner's movements to the other. Mattresses made from memory foam are good options to reduce motion transmission.

2. Try the Scandinavian method: one bed, two duvets or bed covers. If your partner is a sheet-stealer or their kicking or thrashing about leaves you literally in the cold, then you might try the custom used throughout Scandinavia and Germany to have one bed but separate covers for each partner.

3. Twin beds put together as one. Two twins make a king, but you can have separate sheeting for each of you, to minimize

disruption by one person's movements and have a king-size duvet on top, so it still looks like a king-size bed.

4. Ear plugs and white noise machines are good options for blocking or drowning out the noise of a snoring partner.

5. Consider separate beds, particularly if it is a safety issue. But if you go this route, talk about it, and come to a decision together about how you are going to make it work, including strategies to maintain intimacy.

chapter ten

NEGOTIATING THE NIGHT

MELANIE AND CHRIS WERE IN TROUBLE. THEY HAD BEEN MARRIED for five years. And when it came to sleep, they were wired differently. Melanie was a hardcore lark. Chris was an owl's owl. Melanie's ideal bedtime was somewhere between nine and ten at night, and she comfortably would wake up around five thirty a.m., feeling rested and alert. Chris, a guy who worked in tech, had a flexible work schedule (which was a good thing for him), because he felt most productive in the evening hours, and waking up before ten a.m. was to him, akin to torture. They knew this about each other well before they got married, and it wasn't a problem at first, but it became one when they decided to leave their jobs and go into business together to start a digital marketing consultancy. Getting a new business off the ground is a lot of work. It's also stressful. Add to that stress the fact that you're trying to have a business partnership with your life partner, and you're already asking for some trouble. That trouble for Melanie and Chris became amplified because of their differences in sleep.

"There's a lot to get done when you're getting a company off the ground," Melanie said to me. "And I'd just get so frustrated with Chris when I was ready to work and he just wasn't. And then when I was ready to stop working and just be a couple together, that was when he wanted to focus on the work. It was just completely incompatible." Chris agreed, saying, "Yeah, we were out of sync at work, and it was spilling over into our relationship, too. We weren't really being that nice to each other as coworkers or as partners. We definitely weren't spending much time in bed together. It was threatening all of it." Chris would try to force Melanie to stay up late and discuss work stuff while she was ready to wind down. Melanie would schedule early morning client calls, expecting Chris to show up ready to roll, and he'd struggle to engage.

Luckily, they recognized the problem early. They knew they were doing something "nuts" (their words) by going into business together, but they really wanted to make it work. It was a dream they had for a long time. They valued each other's talents and expertise as marketers. They knew they had the stuff to make a great business. They just needed to figure out how to accommodate their individual preferences and needs for how and when they worked, how and when they slept, and how they'd continue to honor the nonwork part of their relationship. They needed to negotiate the night—and the day. And that's what they did.

They sat down and made a plan. They created a system that focused the collaborative parts of their work between ten and three, and the more independent parts of their work were reserved for those parts of the day when each of them worked best—late at night for

Chris, early in the morning for Melanie. They also recognized that they needed to make sure they held sacred the romantic side of their partnership even while trying to foster the professional side, so they both agreed to go to bed together every night just to have some time together to end their day. For Melanie, that would literally end by going to sleep, at which point Chris would often get back up and go knock out a few more things for work. He'd crawl back into their bed afterward, and generally Melanie would be none the wiser. She would wake up while he was still sound asleep, and she'd get up and get some things done before they'd both take a break for a shared breakfast.

Because of their willingness to recognize and acknowledge their problem and come together quickly to create their own shared sleep action plan, I'm happy to report that both of their relationships (their marriage and their business) are going strong.

If all this sounds as if it were a bit too easy or a bit too good to be true, that's because it is. Up to this point, every couple's story I've shared with you is real, and they all reflected just how challenging it can be to figure out their sleep and their relationships and how they wanted them to be. The story of Melanie and Chris is also based on a real couple suffering from real challenges that many couples face. What's not real is the way I made it sound as if they seemingly solved their issues in the course of a night. That's not how it works. Most of us have to struggle for a while with our sleep challenges before we actually do something about it. Most couples don't recognize the outsized role that their sleep might be playing in the quality of their relationship or how the quality of their relationship is affecting their sleep. And for most couples, the work of getting on the same page about all this stuff isn't something that gets cleared up in one dinner table conversation or pillow talk session. So while I wish every couple could be like my somewhat fictionalized couple Melanie and Chris and immediately take action when things start to go south, my years in private practice (and in marriage) make it clear that that's not what usually happens.

But you? Herein lies your opportunity. You and your partner don't have to be most couples. After completing the chapters of this book, you now have a deep understanding of the interconnected nature of sleep quality and relationship quality, and you also have insight into the key practices associated with bolstering both. You understand the importance of recognizing differences in sleep preferences. You have a greater appreciation for the ways that sleep can go wrong and what you can do if it does. You know all the ways that sleep can affect your physical health, mental health, and relationship health, and you recognize how all those things can affect your ability to sleep. You know that the ups and downs and normal transitions of life, like having children, can have an impact on your sleep. And you know that when you sacrifice your sleep, you are sacrificing your ability to be the partners you want to be—that your relationship needs you to be.

I hope you now have the confidence to find the sleeping arrangement that will work best for you and your partner. There are no right or wrong ways when it comes to couples' sleeping arrangements, because there is no one-size-fits-all sleeping strategy. There are, however, lots of wrong ways to approach this topic, and those generally start by basing your decisions on expectations or assumptions, or reacting to the situation, without ever talking about what's working or not working in your coupled sleep experience. By reading this book, if you and your partner have been taking the time to complete your

Shared Sleep Action Plan, you've been doing the work that needs to be done. More than anything this book was designed to help you and your partner open the conversation about a significant and important part of your lives that more often than not people fail to discuss at all. Decisions are too often made implicitly, based on societal beliefs, expectations, and assumptions rather than open and honest communication. That doesn't have to be how things go for you. So while Melanie and Chris may have been a bit of a fairy tale, you now have within you all that you need to create with your partner your very own nonfiction sleep success story.

SHARED SLEEP ACTION PLAN:
Negotiating the Night

For this final installment of your Shared Sleep Action Plan, I want to give you a set of questions to discuss with your partner so you can do what Melanie and Chris did in my fictionalized account. I want to help you negotiate the night. So if you're not already there, crawl in bed together, and work through these few queries. As you do, remember some key ground rules for negotiation within couples:

1. Allow each of you to express what you want from the situation.
2. When expressing your wants and including what you want to change, keep it simple and direct, and stay focused on the topic at hand (for this purpose, on sleep).
3. Listen to your partner.
4. Be in a good place mentally and physically to negotiate— and that includes being well-rested.

Taking such steps is critical to arrive at a mutual set of goals, so both parties, and ultimately the relationship, win.

Question 1: How do you think our relationship would be better if we improved the third of our lives we spend asleep?

Question 2: If you had your way, how would we sleep as a couple? What time would we go to bed? What type of bed would we sleep in (if together)? Would we sleep apart? How important are these things to you?

Question 3: What feels like a reasonable, achievable goal we could have for our sleep? How will we know we've achieved it?

Question 4: Sleep deprivation will happen. What is your partner like when they are slangry? (sleepy + angry = slangry, or sleep deprivation–induced anger.) How does it manifest? What can you do for each other when it is clear that sleep problems are keeping one or both of you from being your best selves? Although it is certainly not an excuse for chronically bad behavior or chronically self-induced sleep deprivation, sometimes putting a label on why you or your partner might be behaving badly can give you that little bit of emotional distance you need to de-escalate a conflict.

Question 5: Research shows that endings are important—end of this book, end of the day. Couples can lose the ritual of closing the day with each other, by distractions, technology, and racing to bed instead of preparing for bed. How can you as a couple make sure that you end every night on a good note, in bed, regardless of whether you both go to sleep? What routine might you establish for ending every night (or at least most nights) right?

EPILOGUE

EARLY IN THIS BOOK I NOTED THAT THE ONE QUESTION I RECEIVE most often is, "Is it bad if my partner and I sleep apart?" Of course, I've thoroughly answered that question. Just to reiterate, whether or not you share a bed says little about your relationship. How you have come to that decision as a couple says a lot more.

A close second most often asked question I get is this: "So do you and your husband sleep together or apart?" Normally, when I get this question, I deflect and say something to the effect of, "My sleeping arrangements are really irrelevant, right?" As a clinician, I have been taught to be cautious and judicious about how much I disclose about myself to clients or others who are seeking my expert opinion. Sometimes, self-disclosure can help build a therapeutic relationship, as such openness can help create a sense of connection between me and whoever is doing the asking. But caution is warranted, because whether in my role as a clinician or as a subject matter expert on the topic, I fear the motivation behind the question is often to derive some sense of validation for one's own behavior. If I say, "My husband and I sleep together," and the person who is asking is contemplating, or has already made the choice, to sleep apart from their partner, then they might feel implicitly judged or worried that they made the wrong decision. On the other hand, if my answer coincides with whatever sleeping arrangement the asker currently has, then that may be taken as tacit agreement that this is necessarily the best or right choice for that couple. How am I to know what works best for a given couple, with such limited knowledge? All that said, since you've borne with me throughout these pages, I will self-disclose just a bit. The answer is (drumroll please): my husband and I share a bed.

If you really want to know the details, it's a king-sized bed. After having kids and as personal space and sleep became increasingly precious, after a lot of discussion (and some resistance from me), we sized up from a queen-size bed to a California king. This hasn't always been easy, and sometimes I regret the decision, because even though we continue to share a bed, albeit a bigger one, I am aware that the extra space afforded us can make it far too easy to sleep separately, even if we're technically sleeping together. Sometimes, particularly when life gets really crazy (and frankly, when we could use each other's physical comfort the most), we fall into a pattern of living parallel and separate lives in bed. Whenever I catch this pattern emerging, however, I literally do the smallest thing. I simply reach over and put my hand on his hand or on his arm or his stomach, and doing so provides this immediate sense of connection and calm.

Epilogue

Whatever your sleeping arrangement, whether cuddled up in a double, spread apart on a California king, or sleeping in separate rooms entirely, it is important to remember the profound importance of touch. It's one of the basic human needs, and skin hunger does exist. In fact, in this era of social distancing and COVID-19, it's taken on increased awareness, given how many are being deprived of that basic human need.

We may assume that skin hunger is primarily the affliction of those living alone, but I'd venture to guess that even the partnered among us self-impose some degree of skin hunger by neglecting to take advantage of the powerful salve of human touch. Maybe sleeping together isn't for everyone, but human touch is essential, and the bed is a great place to do that. So even if you choose not to sleep together, don't forsake the cuddle.

Good night. Sleep tight. Sweet dreams.

Notes

INTRODUCTION: LOVE IN THE AGE OF SLEEPLESSNESS

x   *Consequently, the majority of therapeutic sleep*: Rogojanski J, Carney CE, Monson CM. "Interpersonal factors in insomnia: a model for integrating bed partners into cognitive behavioral therapy for insomnia." *Sleep Medicine Reviews* 2013; 17 (1): 55–64.

xi   *In its annual survey*: 2005 *Sleep in America Poll*. Washington, DC: National Sleep Foundation, 2005.

xii   *women are about twice as likely to have insomnia*: Zhang B, Wing YK. "Sex differences in insomnia: a meta-analysis." *Sleep* 2006; 29 (1): 85–93.

xiii   *In fact, eight out of ten adults*: Graf N. "Key findings on marriage and cohabitation in the U.S." Pew Research Center. November 6, 2019. pewresearch.org/fact-tank/2019/11/06/key -findings-on-marriage-and-cohabitation-in-the-u-s.

xiv   *It's even been said that sleep is the new sex*: Carlson M. "The mummy diaries." *Time* 2002.

xiv   *about one in three American adults regularly*: Krueger PM, Friedman EM. "Sleep duration in the United States: a cross-sectional population-based study." *American Journal of Epidemiology* 2009; 169 (9): 1052–1063.

xv *Sleep loss and sleep disruption are directly linked with increased risk for mental health problems*: Walker MP. *Why We Sleep: Unlocking the Power of Sleep and Dreams.* New York: Scribner, 2017.

xv *sleep loss costs the US economy $411 billion per year*: Hafner M, Stepanek M, Taylor J, Troxel WM, van Stolk C. *Why Sleep Matters—The Economic Costs of Insufficient Sleep: A Cross-Country Comparative Analysis.* Santa Monica, CA: RAND Corporation, 2016.

xix *They say that when China came out of lockdown*: Prasso S. "China's divorce spike is a warning to rest of locked-down world." Bloomberg. March 31, 2020. bloomberg.com/news /articles/2020-03-31/divorces-spike-in-china-after-coronavirus -quarantines.

CHAPTER 1: SLEEPING TOGETHER (OR NOT)

4 *or in the words of journalist*: Goldstein JM. "Sleep divorce is a thing—and it's on the rise." *Washingtonian.* Nov. 5, 2019. washingtonian.com/2019/11/05/sleep-divorce-on-the-rise.

5 *Sleep makes up about one-third of your entire life*: Aminoff MJ, Boller F, Swaab DF. "We spend about one-third of our life either sleeping or attempting to do so." *Handbook of Clinical Neurology* 2011; 98.

6 *Historian A. Roger Ekirch wrote that night was*: Ekirch AR. *At Day's Close: The Night in Times Past.* New York: Norton, 2005.

7 *An Italian proverb advised sleepers*: Torriano G. *Piazza Universale Di Proverbi Italiani, or, A Common Place of Italian Proverbs and Proverbial Phrases.* London: F. and T.W., 1666.

7 *In the 1768 diary entries of John Eliot*: Jerningham M. *The Welch Heiress: A Comedy.* 2nd ed. London: R. White, 1795.

8   *In the words of renowned couples' therapist, Esther Perel*:
Schwartz A. "Esther Perel Lets Us Listen in on Couples' Se-
crets." *The New Yorker* May 31, 2017.

9   *In 1861 an influential doctor, William Whitty*: Hall WW. *Sleep;
or, The Hygiene of the Night*. New York: Hurd and Houghton.
1870.

9   *Hence, the proliferation of twin beds*: Hinds H. *A Cultural History of Twin Beds*. London: Bloomsbury Academic, 2019.

9   *Rules governing what was morally acceptable or unacceptable*:
The Motion Picture Production Code of 1930 (Hays Code).
Arts Reformation. artsreformation.com/a001/hays-code.html.
Accessed July 6, 2020.

10 *In 2007, the National Association of Homebuilders*: Rozhon T.
"To have, hold and cherish, until bedtime." *New York Times*
March 11, 2007.

11 *According to several studies, when sleep is measured*: Dittami J,
Keckeis M, Machatschke I, Katina S, Zeitlhofer J, Kloesch G.
"Sex differences in the reactions to sleeping in pairs versus sleeping alone in humans." *Sleep and Biological Rhythms* 2007; 5
(4): 271–276. Meadows R, Arber S, Venn S, Hislop J, Stanley
N. "Exploring the interdependence of couples' rest-wake cycles:
an actigraphic study." *Chronobiology International* 2009; 26 (1):
80–92. Meadows R, Venn S, Hislop J, Stanley N, Arber S. "In-
vestigating couples' sleep: an evaluation of actigraphic analysis
techniques." *Journal of Sleep Research* 2005; 14 (4): 377–386.
Pankhurst FP, Horne JA. "The influence of bed partners on
movement during sleep." *Sleep* 1994; 17 (4): 308–315.

12 *if you sleep with a snorer*: Beninati W, Harris CD, Herold DL,
Shepard JW. "The effect of snoring and obstructive sleep
apnea on the sleep quality of bed partners." *Mayo Clinic Proceedings* 1999; 74 (10): 955–958.

12 *Given that men are more likely to be snorers*: Dittami J, Keckeis
M, Machatschke I, Katina S, Zeitlhofer J, Kloesch G. "Sex

differences in the reactions to sleeping in pairs versus sleeping alone in humans."

12   *a more recent study suggests sleeping together*: Drews HJ, Wallot S, Brysch P, et al. "Bed-sharing in couples is associated with increased and stabilized REM sleep and sleep-stage synchronization." *Frontiers in Psychiatry* June 25, 2020.

12   *On top of that, when you ask people*: Monroe LJ. "Transient changes in EEG sleep patterns of married good sleepers: the effects of altering sleeping arrangement." *Psychophysiology* 1969; 6 (3): 330–337. Pankhurst FP, Horne JA. "The influence of bed partners on movement during sleep."

16   *The evidence suggests that most adults need*: Hirshkowitz M, Whiton K, Albert SM, et al. "National Sleep Foundation's updated sleep duration recommendations: final report." *Sleep Health* 2015; 1 (4): 233–243.

16   *Studies have shown that there may be health consequences*: Bliwise DL, Young TB. "The parable of parabola: what the U-shaped curve can and cannot tell us about sleep." *Sleep* 2007; 30 (12): 1614–1615.

16   *but there is variability across individuals*: Chaput JP, Dutil C, Sampasa-Kanyinga H. "Sleeping hours: what is the ideal number and how does age impact this?" *Nature and Science of Sleep* 2018; 10: 421–430.

16   *only about 2 percent of the population*: He Y, Jones CR, Fujiki N, et al. "The transcriptional repressor DEC2 regulates sleep length in mammals." *Science* 2009; 325: 866–870.

CHAPTER 2: SLEEP AS IF YOUR RELATIONSHIP DEPENDS ON IT

21   *The renowned relationship expert*: Gottman J. "Predicting the longitudinal course of marriages." *Journal of Marital and Family Therapy* 2007; 17: 3–7. Gottman, JM. *What Predicts*

Divorce? The Relationship Between Marital Processes and Marital Outcomes. Hillsdale, NJ: Erlbaum, 1994. Gottman JM, Coan J, Carrere S, Swanson C. "Predicting marital happiness and stability from newlywed interactions." *Journal of Marriage and the Family* 1998; 60 (1): 5–22.

21   *the Four Horsemen of the Apocalypse*: Gottman J, Silver N. *The Principles for Making Marriage Work: A Practical Guide from the Country's Foremost Relationship Expert.* New York: Three Rivers, 1999.

24   *Sleep plays a powerful role*: Gruber R, Cassoff J. "The interplay between sleep and emotion regulation: conceptual framework empirical evidence and future directions." *Current Psychiatry Reports* 2014; 16 (11): 500. Palmer CA, Alfano CA. "Sleep and emotion regulation: an organizing, integrative review." *Sleep Medicine Reviews* 2017; 31: 6–16.

24   *Studies have shown that when sleep was restricted*: Dinges DF, Pack F, Williams K, et al. "Cumulative sleepiness, mood disturbance, and psychomotor vigilance performance decrements during a week of sleep restricted to 4–5 hours per night." *Sleep* 1997; 20 (4): 267–277.

24   *Research has further shown that sleep loss*: Franzen PL, Siegle GJ, Buysse DJ. "Relationships between affect, vigilance, and sleepiness following sleep deprivation." *Journal of Sleep Research* 2008; 17 (1): 34–41.

24   *Sleep disturbances are a symptom*: Baglioni C, Nanovska S, Regen W, et al. "Sleep and mental disorders: a meta-analysis of polysomnographic research." *Psychological Bulletin* 2016; 142 (9): 969–990.

24   *they exacerbate existing ones*: Krystal AD. "Psychiatric disorders and sleep." *Neurological Clinics* 2012; 30 (4): 1389–1413.

24   *They also can predict the onset*: Baglioni C, Battagliese G, Feige B, et al. "Insomnia as a predictor of depression: a

meta-analytic evaluation of longitudinal epidemiological studies." *Journal of Affective Disorders* 2011; 135 (1–3): 10–19. Lin H-T, Lai C-H, Perng H-J, et al. "Insomnia as an independent predictor of suicide attempts: a nationwide population-based retrospective cohort study." *BMC Psychiatry* 2018; 18 (1): 117. Shanahan L, Copeland WE, Angold A, Bondy CL, Costello EJ. "Sleep problems predict and are predicted by generalized anxiety/depression and oppositional defiant disorder." *Journal of the American Academy of Child and Adolescent Psychiatry* 2014; 53 (5): 550–558.

24 *Left untreated, sleep problems predict*: Troxel WM, Kupfer DJ, Reynolds CF 3rd, et al. "Insomnia and objectively measured sleep disturbances predict treatment outcome in depressed patients treated with psychotherapy or psychotherapy-pharmacotherapy combinations." *Journal of Clinical Psychiatry* 2012; 73 (4): 478–485. Franzen PL, Buysse DJ. "Sleep disturbances and depression: risk relationships for subsequent depression and therapeutic implications." *Dialogues in Clinical Neuroscience* 2008; 10 (4): 473–481.

24 *For example, a multinational study*: Breslau J, Miller E, Jin R, et al. "A multinational study of mental disorders, marriage, and divorce." *Acta Psychiatrica Scandinavica* 2011; 124 (6): 474–486.

25 *Under sleep-deprived conditions, people show activation*: van der Helm E, Walker MP. "Sleep and affective brain regulation." *Social and Personality Psychology Compass* 2012; 6 (11): 773–791.

25 *also show a dampening of response*: Krause AJ, Simon EB, Mander BA, et al. "The sleep-deprived human brain." *Nature Reviews Neuroscience* 2017; 18 (7): 404–418.

25 *The more sleep-deprived we become*: Van Dongen HP, Maislin G, Mullington JM, Dinges DF. "The cumulative cost of additional wakefulness: dose-response effects on neurobehavioral functions and sleep physiology from chronic sleep

restriction and total sleep deprivation." *Sleep* 2003; 26 (2): 117–126.

25 *Decades of relationship research:* Overall NC, McNulty JK. "What type of communication during conflict is beneficial for intimate relationships?" *Current Opinion in Psychology* 2017; 13: 1–5.

26 *They found that on nights when couples slept worse:* Gordon AM, Chen S. "The role of sleep in interpersonal conflict: do sleepless nights mean worse fights?" *Social Psychology and Personality Science* 2013; 5 (2): 168–175.

26 *As Dr. Gordon explains it:* Amie Gordon, personal communication, July 12, 2019.

26 *Researchers at the Ohio State University:* Wilson SJ, Jaremka LM, Fagundes CP, et al. "Shortened sleep fuels inflammatory responses to marital conflict: emotion regulation matters." *Psychoneuroendocrinology* 2017; 79: 74–83.

27 *Author, public speaker, and professor of social work:* Brown B. *Daring Greatly: How the Courage to Be Vulnerable Transforms the Way We Live, Love, Parent, and Lead.* New York: Gotham, 2012.

27 *research suggests that genuine expressions of empathy:* "Empathic accuracy." Psychology. psychology.iresearchnet.com /social-psychology/interpersonal-relationships/empathic -accuracy. Accessed September 9, 2020.

28 *Drs. Gordon and Chen found not only:* Gordon AM, Chen S. "The role of sleep in interpersonal conflict."

28 *Psychologist Eleanor McGlinchey used:* McGlinchey EL, Talbot LS, Chang K-h, Kaplan KA, Dahl RE, Harvey AG. "The effect of sleep deprivation on vocal expression of emotion in adolescents and adults." *Sleep* 2011; 34 (9): 1233–1241.

29 *Industrial-organizational psychologists who study:* Patterson K, Grenny J, McMillan R, Switzler A. *Crucial Conversations: Tools for Talking When Stakes Are High.* New York: McGraw-Hill, 2011.

30   *Studies have shown that under sleep-deprived conditions, decision making*: Killgore WD, Balkin TJ, Wesensten NJ. "Impaired decision making following 49 h of sleep deprivation." *Journal of Sleep Research* 2006; 15 (1): 7–13.

30   *We are more distracted and more prone to risky*: Harrison Y, Horne JA. "The impact of sleep deprivation on decision making: a review." *Journal of Experimental Psychology: Applied.* 2000; 6 (3): 236–249.

30   *Researchers at Walter Reed Army Research Institute*: Killgore WD, Lipizzi EL, Kamimori GH, Balkin TJ. "Caffeine effects on risky decision making after 75 hours of sleep deprivation." *Aviation, Space, and Environmental Medicine* 2007; 78 (10): 957–962.

30   *Those same researchers at Walter Reed*: Killgore WD, Killgore DB, Day LM, Li C, Kamimori GH, Balkin TJ. "The effects of 53 hours of sleep deprivation on moral judgment." *Sleep* 2007; 30 (3): 345–352.

31   *Science tells us that social isolation*: Klinenberg E. "Social isolation, loneliness, and living alone: identifying the risks for public health." *American Journal of Public Health* 2016; 106 (5): 786–787.

31   *In a series of elegant studies published in 2018*: Ben Simon E, Walker MP. "Sleep loss causes social withdrawal and loneliness." *Nature Communications* 2018; 9 (1): 3146.

33   *a University of Michigan study of women's sleep patterns*: Kalmbach DA, Arnedt JT, Pillai V, Ciesla JA. "The impact of sleep on female sexual response and behavior: a pilot study." *Journal of Sexual Medicine* 2015; 12 (5): 1221–1232.

33   *A 2011 study published in the preeminent*: Leproult R, Van Cauter E. "Effect of 1 week of sleep restriction on testosterone levels in young healthy men." *Journal of the American Medical Association* 2011; 305 (21): 2173–2174.

34   *A more recent study showed a positive, linear relationship*: Zhang W, Piotrowska K, Chavoshan B, Wallace J, Liu PY. "Sleep duration is associated with testis size in healthy young men." *Journal of Clinical Sleep Medicine* 2018; 14 (10): 1757–1764.

36   *My research has shown that sleep loss affects relationships*: Hasler BP, Troxel WM. "Couples' nighttime sleep efficiency and concordance: evidence for bidirectional associations with daytime relationship functioning." *Psychosomatic Medicine* 2010; 72 (8): 794–801.

CHAPTER 3: A TOXIC DANCE

46   *sleep loss can compromise immune functioning*: Prather AA, Janicki-Deverts D, Hall MH, Cohen S. "Behaviorally assessed sleep and susceptibility to the common cold." *Sleep* 2015; 38 (9): 1353–1359.

46   *happily married or partnered people have lower rates of depression*: Bulloch AG, Williams JV, Lavorato DH, Patten SB. "The relationship between major depression and marital disruption is bidirectional." *Depression and Anxiety* 2009; 26 (12): 1172–1177. Robards J, Evandrou M, Falkingham J, Vlachantoni A. "Marital status, health and mortality." *Maturitas* 2012; 73 (4): 295–299. Schoenborn CA. "Marital status and health: United States, 1999–2002." *Advance Data* 2004; 351. Wong CW, Kwok CS, Narain A, et al. "Marital status and risk of cardiovascular diseases: a systematic review and meta-analysis." *Heart* 2018; 104: 1937–1948.

47   *On the other hand, a high-quality relationship may buffer*: Troxel WM, Robles TF, Hall M, Buysse DJ. "Marital quality and the marital bed: examining the covariation between relationship quality and sleep." *Sleep Medicine Reviews* 2007; 11 (5): 389–404.

47 *In 2001, researchers from the Ohio State University*: Kiecolt-Glaser JK, Newton TL. "Marriage and health: his and hers." *Psychological Bulletin* 2001; 127 (4): 472–503.

48 *In the past two decades following the article's publication*: Robles TF, Slatcher RB, Trombello JM, McGinn MM. "Marital quality and health: a meta-analytic review." *Psychological Bulletin* 2014; 140 (1): 140–187.

48 *And sure enough, what we and others have found*: Gallo LC, Troxel WM, Matthews KA, Kuller LH. "Marital status and quality in middle-aged women: Associations with levels and trajectories of cardiovascular risk factors." *Health Psychology* 2003; 22 (5): 453–463. Robles TF. "Marital quality and health: implications for marriage in the 21st century." *Current Directions in Psychological Science* 2014; 23 (6): 427–432. Troxel WM, Matthews KA, Gallo LC, Kuller LH. "Marital quality and occurrence of the metabolic syndrome in women." *Archives of Internal Medicine* 2005; 165 (9): 1022–1027.

49 *For example, when we studied maried, heterosexual couples' sleep*: Hasler BP, Troxel WM. "Couples' nighttime sleep efficiency and concordance: evidence for bidirectional associations with daytime relationship functioning." *Psychosomatic Medicine* 2010; 72 (8): 794–801.

50 *It is in our DNA to depend on our social connections*: Robinson GE, Fernald RD, Clayton DF. "Genes and social behavior." *Science* 2008; 322 (5903): 896–900.

50 *having a high level of attachment anxiety*: Maunder RG, Hunter JJ, Lancee WJ. "The impact of attachment insecurity and sleep disturbance on symptoms and sick days in hospital-based health-care workers." *Journal of Psychosomatic Research* 2011; 70 (1): 11–17. Niko Verdecias R, Jean-Louis G, Zizi F, Casimir GJ, Browne RC. "Attachment styles and sleep measures in a community-based sample of older adults." *Sleep*

Medicine 2009; 10 (6): 664–667. Troxel WM, Cyranowski JM, Hall M, Frank E, Buysse DJ. "Attachment anxiety, relationship context, and sleep in women with recurrent major depression." *Psychosomatic Medicine* 2007; 69 (7) 692–699. Troxel WM, Germain A. "Insecure attachment is an independent correlate of objective sleep disturbances in military veterans." *Sleep Medicine* 2011; 12 (9): 860–865.

50 *victims of domestic violence experience high levels*: El-Sheikh M, Kelly RJ, Koss KJ, Rauer AJ. "Longitudinal relations between constructive and destructive conflict and couples' sleep." *Journal of Family Psychology* 2015; 29 (3): 349–359. Pigeon WR, Cerulli C, Richards H, He H, Perlis M, Caine E. "Sleep disturbances and their association with mental health among women exposed to intimate partner violence." *Journal of Women's Health* 2011; 20 (12): 1923–1929. Rauer AJ, Kelly RJ, Buckhalt JA, El-Sheikh M. "Sleeping with one eye open: marital abuse as an antecedent of poor sleep." *Journal of Family Psychology* 2010; 24 (6): 667–677.

50 *Furthermore, even among victims who leave their abuser*: Matos M, Gonçalves M. "Sleep and women intimate partner victimization: prevalence, effects and good practices in health care settings." *Sleep Science* 2019; 12 (1): 35–42.

51 *Research has shown that couples who were able to share*: Kane HS, Slatcher RB, Reynolds BM, Repetti RL, Robles TF. "Daily self-disclosure and sleep in couples." *Health Psychology* 2014; 33 (8): 813–822.

51 *Another such behavior is practicing gratitude*: Gordon AM, Chen S. "Too tired to say thanks? a multi-method investigation of sleep and gratitude." Paper presented at the annual meeting of the Society for Personality and Social Psychology, New Orleans. January 2013. Lambert NM, Fincham FD. "Expressing gratitude to a partner leads to more relationship maintenance behavior." *Emotion* 2011; 11 (1): 52–60.

52 *Being in a healthy relationship is also beneficial*: Leach LS, Butterworth P, Olesen SC, Mackinnon A. "Relationship quality and levels of depression and anxiety in a large population-based survey." *Social Psychiatry and Psychiatric Epidemiology* 2012; 48: 417–425. Proulx CM, Helms HM, Buehler C. "Marital quality and personal well-being: a meta-analysis." *Journal of Marriage and Family* 2007; 69: 576–593.

52 *These incessant and intrusive thoughts*: Lancee J, Eisma MC, van Zanten KB, Topper M. "When thinking impairs sleep: trait, daytime and nighttime repetitive thinking in insomnia." *Behavioral Sleep Medicine* 2017; 15 (1): 53–69.

52 *Being depressed increases your risk*: Rajan S, McKee M, Rangarajan S, et al. "Association of symptoms of depression with cardiovascular disease and mortality in low-, middle-, and high-income countries." *JAMA Psychiatry* June 10, 2020.

53 *depression has joined the ranks*: Freedland KE, Carney RM. "Depression as a risk factor for adverse outcomes in coronary heart disease." *BMC Medicine* 2013; 11: 131.

53 *Scientists call this "social control."*: Lewis MA, Rook KS. "Social control in personal relationships: impact on health behaviors and psychological distress." *Health Psychology* 1999; 18: 63–71.

53 *This type of influence by one's partner can be*: Rook KS, Zettel LA. "The purported benefits of marriage viewed through the lens of physical health." *Psychological Inquiry* 2005; 16: 116–121.

54 *Our research has shown that for a woman*: Hasler BP, Troxel WM. "Couples' nighttime sleep efficiency and concordance."

54 *Scientists who study circadian rhythms use the German word*: Ehlers CL, Frank E, Kupfer DJ. "Social zeitgebers and biological rhythms." *Archives of General Psychiatry* 1988; 45 (10): 948–952.

55 *The fight-or-flight response involves*: McEwen, BS. "Physiology and neurobiology of stress and adaptation: central role of the brain." *Physiological Reviews* 2007; 87: 873–904.

56   *In one of my favorite studies of all time*: Kiecolt-Glaser JK, Loving TJ, Stowell JR, et al. "Hostile marital interactions, proinflammatory cytokine production, and wound healing." *Archives of General Psychiatry* 2005; 62 (12): 1377–1384.

56   *In a subsequent study*: Wilson SJ, Jaremka LM, Fagundes CP, et al. "Shortened sleep fuels inflammatory responses to marital conflict: emotion regulation matters." *Psychoneuroendocrinology* 2017; 79: 74–83.

57   *Oxytocin is a hormone produced in the brain*: Algoe SB, Kurtz LE, Grewen K. "Oxytocin and social bonds: the role of oxytocin in perceptions of romantic partners' bonding behavior." *Psychological Science* 2017; 28 (12): 1763–1772.

57   *The release of oxytocin*: Sippel LM, Allington CE, Pietrzak RH, Harpaz-Rotem I, Mayes LC, Olff M. "Oxytocin and stress-related disorders: neurobiological mechanisms and treatment opportunities." *Chronic Stress* 2017; 1: 2470547016687996.

57   *However, there is strikingly little research*: Lancel M, Krömer S, Neumann ID. "Intracerebral oxytocin modulates sleep-wake behaviour in male rats." *Regulatory Peptides* 2003; 114 (2–3): 145–152.

57   *In an Australian study*: Lastella M, O'Mullan C, Paterson JL, Reynolds AC. "Sex and sleep: perceptions of sex as a sleep promoting behavior in the general adult population." *Frontiers in Public Health* 2019; 7: 33.

58   *At this point, only a handful of studies*: Fekete EM, Seay J, Antoni MH, et al. "Oxytocin, social support, and sleep quality in low-income minority women living with HIV." *Behavioral Sleep Medicine* 2014; 12 (3) 207–221. Jain V, Marbach J, Kimbro S, et al. "Benefits of oxytocin administration in obstructive sleep apnea." *American Journal of Physiology—Lung Cellular and Molecular Physiology* 2017; 313 (5): L825–L833. Schuh-Hofer S, Eichhorn N, Grinevich V,

Treede RD. "Sleep deprivation related changes of plasma oxytocin in males and female contraceptive users depend on sex and correlate differentially with anxiety and pain hypersensitivity." *Frontiers in Behavioral Neuroscience* 2018; 12: 161.

59   *Sleep, like virtually every other health outcome*: Egan KJ, Knutson KL, Pereira AC, von Schantz M. "The role of race and ethnicity in sleep, circadian rhythms and cardiovascular health." *Sleep Medicine Reviews* 2017; 33: 70–78. Hale L. "Who has time to sleep?" *Journal of Public Health* 2005; 27 (2): 205–211. Hale L, Troxel W, Buysse DJ. "Sleep health: an opportunity for public health to address health equity." *Annual Review of Public Health* 2020; 41 (1): 81–99. Jackson CL, Redline S, Kawachi I, Williams MA, Hu FB. "Racial disparities in short sleep duration by occupation and industry." *American Journal of Epidemiology* 2013; 178 (9): 1442–1451.

59   *Substantial research shows that where people live*: Auchincloss AH, Diez Roux AV, Mujahid MS, Shen M, Bertoni AG, Carnethon MR. "Neighborhood resources for physical activity and healthy foods and incidence of type 2 diabetes mellitus: the multi-ethnic study of atherosclerosis." *Archives of Internal Medicine* 2009; 169 (18): 1698–1704. Diez-Roux AV. *Neighborhoods and Health*. 2nd ed. New York: Oxford University Press, 2018. Hale L, Hill TD, Friedman E, et al. "Perceived neighborhood quality, sleep quality, and health status: evidence from the Survey of the Health of Wisconsin." *Social Science & Medicine* 2013; 79: 16–22.

CHAPTER 4: A VIRTUOUS CYCLE

65   *Swedish researchers showed subjects photos*: Sundelin T, Lekander M, Sorjonen K, Axelsson J. "Negative effects of restricted sleep on facial appearance and social appeal." *Royal Society Open Science* 2017; 4 (5): 160918.

65 *Another study by University of Michigan*: Chervin RD, Ruz-
icka DL, Vahabzadeh A, Burns MC, Burns JW, Buchman
SR. "The face of sleepiness: improvement in appearance after
treatment of sleep apnea." *Journal of Clinical Sleep Medicine*
2013; 9 (9): 845–852.

66 *sleep loss can contribute to expanding*: Patel SR, Hu FB. "Short
sleep duration and weight gain: a systematic review." *Obesity*
2008; 16 (3): 643–653.

66 *People who don't sleep enough or who have poor quality*: Bron-
del L, Romer MA, Nougues PM, Touyarou P, Davenne D.
"Acute partial sleep deprivation increases food intake in
healthy men." *American Journal of Clinical Nutrition* 2010; 91
(6): 1550–1559. Greer SM, Goldstein AN, Walker MP. "The
impact of sleep deprivation on food desire in the human brain."
Nature Communications 2013; 4: 2259. Theorell-Haglöw J,
Lemming EW, Michaëlsson K, Elmståhl S, Lind L, Lindberg
E. "Sleep duration is associated with healthy diet scores and
meal patterns: results from the population-based EpiHealth
study." *Journal of Clinical Sleep Medicine* 2020; 16 (1): 9–18.

66 *In short, according to Gottman and his team's*: Gottman J,
Coan J, Carrere S, Swanson C. "Predicting marital happiness
and stability from newlywed interactions." *Journal of Marriage
and Family* 1998; 60 (1): 5–22.

67 *The slow or "gentle start-up" technique*: Gottman JM, Gottman
JS. "Gottman method couple therapy." In Gurman AS, ed.,
Clinical Handbook of Couple Therapy. New York: Guilford,
2008. 138–164.

68 *Getting the sleep we need also supports our ability*: Watling J,
Pawlik B, Scott K, Booth S, Short MA. "Sleep loss and affective
functioning: more than just mood." *Behavioral Sleep Medicine*
2017; 15 (5): 394–409.

68 *In one study participants reported on a number*: Mauss IB, Troy
AS, LeBourgeois MK. "Poorer sleep quality is associated with

lower emotion-regulation ability in a laboratory paradigm." *Cognition and Emotion* 2013; 27 (3): 567–576.

69   *Cognitive reappraisal is also an important strategy*: Mazzuca S, Kafetsios K, Livi S, Presaghi F. "Emotion regulation and satisfaction in long-term marital relationships: the role of emotional contagion." *Journal of Social and Personal Relationships* 2019; 36 (9): 2880–2895.

69   *Contempt, which may include sarcasm*: Gottman JM. *What Predicts Divorce?* Hillsdale, NJ: Erlbaum Associates, 1994.

70   *Research has shown that couples who slept better*: Gordon AM, Chen S. "Too tired to say thanks? a multi-method investigation of sleep and gratitude." Paper presented at the annual meeting of the Society for Personality and Social Psychology, New Orleans. January 2013.

71   *Jeffrey Hall, a professor of communication studies*: Hall J. "Sexual selection and humor in courtship: a case for warmth and extroversion." *Evolutionary Psychology* 2015; 13 (3): 1–11.

71   *In fact, humor is cited as one of the most valued*: Horn AB, Samson AC, Debrot A, Perrez M. "Positive humor in couples as interpersonal emotion regulation: a dyadic study in everyday life on the mediating role of psychological intimacy." *Journal of Social and Personal Relationships* 2019; 36 (8): 2376–2396.

71   *A study from Walter Reed*: Killgore WD, McBride SA, Killgore DB, Balkin TJ. "The effects of caffeine, dextroamphetamine, and modafinil on humor appreciation during sleep deprivation." *Sleep* 2006; 29 (6): 841–847.

72   *According to a study of more than 170 women*: Kalmbach DA, Arnedt JT, Pillai V, Ciesla JA. "The impact of sleep on female sexual response and behavior: a pilot study." *Journal of Sex Medicine* 2015; 12 (5): 1221–1232.

73   *Research has shown that getting adequate duration*: Gordon AM, Chen S. "The role of sleep in interpersonal conflict: do sleepless

nights mean worse fights?" *Social Psychological and Personality Science* 2013; 5 (2): 168–175. Guadagni V, Burles F, Ferrara M, Iaria G. "The effects of sleep deprivation on emotional empathy." *Journal of Sleep Research* 2014; 23 (6): 657–663.

73   *Research has shown that while healthy sleep can't turn you*: Ben Simon E, Vallat R, Barnes CM, Walker MP. "Sleep loss and the socio-emotional brain." *Trends in Cognitive Science* 2020; 24 (6): 435–450.

73   *Because sleep loss is experienced as a threat*: Prather AA, Bogdan R, Hariri AR. "Impact of sleep quality on amygdala reactivity, negative affect, and perceived stress." *Psychosomatic Medicine* 2013; 75 (4): 350–358. Zenses AK, Lenaert B, Peigneux P, Beckers T, Boddez Y. "Sleep deprivation increases threat beliefs in human fear conditioning." *Journal of Sleep Research* 2020; 29 (3): e12873.

74   *The flooding of emotions and physiological reactivity*: Christensen A. "Dysfunctional interaction patterns in couples." In Noller P, Fitzpatrick MA, eds. *Perspectives on Marital Interaction*. Clevedon, UK: Multilingual Matters, 1988. 31–52. Papp LM, Kouros CD, Cummings EM. "Demand-withdraw patterns in marital conflict in the home." *Personal Relationships* 2009; 16 (2): 285–300.

74   *A team of scientists from the University of California*: Walker MP, van der Helm E. "Overnight therapy? The role of sleep in emotional brain processing." *Psychological Bulletin* 2009; 135 (5): 731–748.

74   *In Gottman's early work*: Gottman JM. *What Predicts Divorce?*

75   *Sleep deprivation and sleep problems*: Basta M, Chrousos GP, Vela-Bueno A, Vgontzas AN. "Chronic insomnia and stress system." *Sleep Medicine Clinics* 2007; 2 (2): 279–291. Franzen PL, Gianaros PJ, Marsland AL, et al. "Cardiovascular reactivity to acute psychological stress following sleep deprivation." *Psychosomatic Medicine* 2011; 73 (8): 679–682.

76 *In 2011, researchers from the University of Utah*: Hicks AM, Diamond LM. "Don't go to bed angry: attachment, conflict, and affective and physiological reactivity." *Personal Relationships* 2011; 18: 266–284.

76 *This is good news for couples*: Gottman J, Dollard C. "Five myths about marriage." *Washington Post* June 1, 2018.

78 *As we sleep, our body temperatures*: Togo F, Aizawa S, Arai J, et al. "Influence on human sleep patterns of lowering and delaying the minimum core body temperature by slow changes in the thermal environment." *Sleep* 2007; 30 (6): 797–802.

79 *Light in general*: Tähkämö L, Partonen T, Pesonen AK. "Systematic review of light exposure impact on human circadian rhythm." *Chronobiology International* 2019; 36 (2): 151–170.

CHAPTER 5: HIS, HERS, AND OUR SLEEP

82 *men are about twice as likely to be snorers*: Chan C, Wong BM, Tang J, et al. "Gender difference in snoring and how it changes with age: systematic review and meta-regression." *Sleep and Breathing* 2012; 16: 977–986.

82 *Women, on the other hand, are more likely to suffer*: Zhang J, Chan NY, Lam SP, et al. "Emergence of sex differences in insomnia symptoms in adolescents: a large-scale school-based study." *Sleep* 2016; 39 (8): 1563–1570.

83 *Sleep researchers refer to these habits*: Irish LA, Kline CE, Gunn HE, Buysse DJ, Hall MH. "The role of sleep hygiene in promoting public health: a review of empirical evidence." *Sleep Medicine Reviews* 2015; 22: 23–36.

83 *There's evidence to suggest*: Dautovich ND, McNamara J, Williams JM, Cross NJ, McCrae CS. "Tackling sleeplessness: psychological treatment options for insomnia." *Nature and Science of Sleep* 2010; 2: 23–37. Jansson-Fröjmark M, Evander J, Alfonsson S. "Are sleep hygiene practices related to the inci-

dence, persistence and remission of insomnia? findings from a prospective community study." *Journal of Behavioral Medicine* 2019; 42 (1): 128–138.

87 *a team of Italian researchers*: Ferrara M, Bottasso A, Tempesta D, Carrieri M, De Gennaro L, Ponti G. "Gender differences in sleep deprivation effects on risk and inequality aversion: evidence from an economic experiment." *PLoS One* 2015; 10 (3): e0120029.

88 *men are two to three times more likely to have the clinical disorder*: Young T, Palta M, Dempsey J, et al. "The occurrence of sleep-disordered breathing among middle-aged adults." *New England Journal of Medicine* 1993; 328: 1230–1235.

88 *Snoring, when it is a symptom of OSA*: Dorasamy P. "Obstructive sleep apnea and cardiovascular risk." *Therapeutics and Clinical Risk Management* 2007; 3 (6): 1105–1111.

88 *Anatomically, men tend to have narrower*: Lin CM, Davidson TM, Ancoli-Israel S. "Gender differences in obstructive sleep apnea and treatment implications." *Sleep Medicine Reviews* 2008; 12 (6): 481–496.

88 *In fact, college and professional football players*: Peck B, Renzi T, Peach H, Gaultney J, Marino JS. "Examination of risk for sleep-disordered breathing among college football players." *Journal of Sport Rehabilitation* 2019; 28 (2): 126–132. Rice TB, Dunn RE, Lincoln AE, et al. "Sleep-disordered breathing in the National Football League." *Sleep* 2010; 33 (6): 819–824.

88 *When airways are narrow*: Eckert DJ, Malhotra A. "Pathophysiology of adult obstructive sleep apnea." *Proceedings of the American Thoracic Society* 2008; 5 (2): 144–153.

88 *Men are more likely to use alcohol: Results from the 2007 National Survey on Drug Use and Health: National Findings*. NSDUH Series H-34, DHHS Publication No. SMA 08-4343. Substance Abuse and Mental Health Services Administration, Office of Applied Studies. Rockville, MD. 2008.

88   *Alcohol can cause the muscles*: Simou E, Britton J, Leonardi-Bee J. "Alcohol and the risk of sleep apnoea: a systematic review and meta-analysis." *Sleep Medicine* 2018; 42: 38–46.

89   *Smoking, too, is statistically more common*: Higgins ST, Kurti AN, Redner R, et al. "A literature review on prevalence of gender differences and intersections with other vulnerabilities to tobacco use in the United States, 2004–2014." *Preventive Medicine* 2015; 80: 89–100.

89   *smoking can cause inflammation in the airways*: Krishnan V, Dixon-Williams S, Thornton JD. "Where there is smoke . . . there is sleep apnea: exploring the relationship between smoking and sleep apnea." *Chest* 2014; 146 (6): 1673–1680.

89   *In the US, as a society as a whole*: Flegal KM, Carroll MD, Ogden CL, Curtin LR. "Prevalence and trends in obesity among US adults, 1999–2008." *Journal of the American Medical Association* 2010; 303 (3): 235–241.

89   *men are more likely than women to carry*: Lin CM, Davidson TM, Ancoli-Israel S. "Gender differences in obstructive sleep apnea and treatment implications." *Sleep Medicine Reviews* 2008; 12 (6): 481–496.

89   *As I mentioned before*: Mallampalli MP, Carter CL. "Exploring sex and gender differences in sleep health: a Society for Women's Health research report." *Journal of Women's Health* 2014; 23 (7): 553–562.

89   *Women are also at greater risk*: Manconi M, Ulfberg J, Berger K, et al. "When gender matters: restless legs syndrome. Report of the 'RLS and woman' workshop endorsed by the European RLS Study Group." *Sleep Medicine Reviews* 2012; 16 (4): 297–307.

90   *For example, women's risk of insomnia*: Nowakowski S, Meers J, Heimbach E. "Sleep and women's health." *Sleep Medicine Research* 2013; 4 (1): 1–22.

90   *significant uptick in sleep problems among women*: Baker FC, Lampio L, Saaresranta T, Polo-Kantola P. "Sleep and sleep

disorders in the menopausal transition." *Sleep Medicine Clinics* 2018; 13 (3): 443–456.

90   *sleep complaints are one of the most common symptoms*: Mong JA, Cusmano DM. "Sex differences in sleep: impact of biological sex and sex steroids." *Philosophical Transactions of the Royal Society B* 2016; 371: 20150110.

91   *we don't see the same steep declines in sleep quality*: Baker FC, de Zambotti M, Colrain IM, Bei B. "Sleep problems during the menopausal transition: prevalence, impact, and management challenges." *Nature and Science of Sleep* 2018; 10: 73–95.

91   *women actually sleep longer and more deeply*: Bixler EO, Papaliaga MN, Vgontzas AN, et al. "Women sleep objectively better than men and the sleep of young women is more resilient to external stressors: effects of age and menopause." *Journal of Sleep Research* 2009; 18: 221–228.

91   *When a more nuanced measurement of sleep*: Buysse DJ, Germain A, Hall ML, et al. "EEG spectral analysis in primary insomnia: NREM period effects and sex differences." *Sleep* 2008; 31 (12): 1673–1682. Mong JA, Cusmano DM. "Sex differences in sleep."

94   *Women, in their study, slept on average*: Burgard SA, Ailshire JA. "Gender and time for sleep among US adults." *American Sociological Review* 2013; 78 (1): 51–69.

CHAPTER 6: ROOM FOR MORE?

103   *In the wake of the 9/11*: Rubenstein LS, Xenakis SN. "Roles of CIA physicians in enhanced interrogation and torture of detainees." *Journal of the American Medical Association* 2010; 304 (5): 569–570.

103   *Although there is ongoing debate*: Seyffert M, Berofsky-Seyffert A. "Waking up to the forensic and ethics risks of systematic

sleep deprivation." *Journal of the American Academy of Psychiatry Law* 2015; 43 (2): 132–136.

107   *Sociologist Rob Meadows*: Meadows RAL. "The negotiated night: an embodied conceptual framework for the sociological study of sleep." *Sociological Review* 2005; 53 (2): 240–254.

107   *In one study, mothers of infants*: Insana SP, Montgomery-Downs HE. "Sleep and sleepiness among first-time postpartum parents: a field- and laboratory-based multimethod assessment." *Developmental Psychobiology* 2013; 55 (4): 361–372.

108   *What's worse is that for mothers*: Insana SP, Williams KB, Montgomery-Downs HE. "Sleep disturbance and neurobehavioral performance among postpartum women." *Sleep* 2013; 36 (1): 73–81.

108   *In fact, research has shown that nearly half*: Insana SP, Williams KB, Montgomery-Downs HE. "Sleep disturbance and neurobehavioral performance."

108   *Studies show that mothers with disturbed sleep*: Goyal D, Gay C, Lee K. "Fragmented maternal sleep is more strongly correlated with depressive symptoms than infant temperament at three months postpartum." *Archives of Women's Mental Health* 2009; 12 (4): 229–237. Tikotzky L, Chambers AS, Kent J, Gaylor E, Manber R. "Postpartum maternal sleep and mothers' perceptions of their attachment relationship with the infant among women with a history of depression during pregnancy." *International Journal of Behavioral Development* 2012; 36 (6): 440–448. Tsai S-Y, Thomas KA. "Sleep disturbances and depressive symptoms in healthy postpartum women: a pilot study." *Research in Nursing & Health* 2012; 35 (3): 314–323.

109   *promising evidence suggests that paying back*: Milner CE, Cote KA. "Benefits of napping in healthy adults: impact of nap length, time of day, age, and experience with napping." *Journal of Sleep Research* 2009; 18 (2): 272–281. Takahashi M.

"The role of prescribed napping in sleep medicine." *Sleep Medicine Reviews* 2003; 7 (3): 227–235.

109 *Research has also shown that mothers*: Ronzio CR, Huntley E, Monaghan M. "Postpartum mothers' napping and improved cognitive growth fostering of infants: results from a pilot study." *Behavioral Sleep Medicine* 2012; 11: 120–132.

109 *In another study, mothers who napped*: Goyal D, Gay C, Lee K. "Fragmented maternal sleep is more strongly correlated with depressive symptoms than infant temperament at three months postpartum." *Archives of Women's Mental Health* 2009; 12 (4): 229–237.

109 *In other words, it's possible*: Cottrell L, Karraker KH. "Correlates of nap taking in mothers of young infants." *Journal of Sleep Research* 2002; 11 (3): 209–212.

110 *Caffeine is the most widely consumed drug*: Evans J, Richards JR, Battisti AS. "Caffeine." StatPearls. March 22, 2020. ncbi .nlm.nih.gov/books/NBK519490.

110 *Breastfeeding moms should exercise caution*: "Caffeine." Drugs and Lactation Database (LactMed). National Library of Medicine. 2006. ncbi.nlm.nih.gov/books/NBK501467.

110 *However, a well-timed cup of coffee*: Institute of Medicine Committee on Military Nutrition Research. "Doses and delivery mechanisms." In *Caffeine for the Sustainment of Mental Task Performance: Formulations for Military Operations*. Washington, DC: National Academies Press, 2001.

110 *And it's always a good idea to talk*: Morgan S, Koren G, Bozzo P. "Is caffeine consumption safe during pregnancy?" *Canadian Family Physician* 2013; 59 (4): 361–362.

111 *Don't fall into the trap*: Hislop J, Arber S. "Sleepers wake! the gendered nature of sleep disruption among mid-life women." *Sociology* 2003; 37 (4): 695–711. Meadows R. "The 'negotiated night': an embodied conceptual framework for the sociological study of sleep." *Sociological Review* 2005; 53: 240–254.

113   *The current guidance*: Task Force on Sudden Infant Death Syndrome. "SIDS and other sleep-related infant deaths: updated 2016 recommendations for a safe infant sleeping environment." *Pediatrics* 2016; 138 (5): e20162938.

113   *And the truth is that many families*: Willinger M, Ko CW, Hoffman HJ, Kessler RC, Corwin MJ. "Trends in infant bed sharing in the United States, 1993–2000: the National Infant Sleep Position study." *Archives of Pediatric and Adolescent Medicine* 2003; 157: 43–49.

114   *attachment parenting*: Sears W, Sears M. *The Attachment Parenting Book: A Commonsense Guide to Understanding and Nurturing Your Baby*. Boston: Little, Brown, 2001.

114   *A substantial amount of research*: Miller P, Commons M. "The benefits of attachment parenting for infants and children: a behavioral developmental view." *Behavioral Development Bulletin* 2016; 10: 1–14.

115   *In fact, one of the most recommended*: Mindell JA, Kuhn B, Lewin DS, Meltzer LJ, Sadeh A, American Academy of Sleep Medicine. "Behavioral treatment of bedtime problems and night wakings in infants and young children." *Sleep* 2006; 29 (10): 1263–1276. Published correction appears in *Sleep* 2006; 29 (11): 1380.

116   *Research shows that when couples are not*: Teti DM, Shimizu M, Crosby B, Kim BR. "Sleep arrangements, parent-infant sleep during the first year, and family functioning." *Developmental Psychology* 2016; 52 (8): 1169–1181.

CHAPTER 7: ARE WE IN SYNC?

121   *most teenagers show a biologically driven "phase delay"*: Carskadon MA. "Sleep in adolescents: the perfect storm." *Pediatric Clinics of North America* 2011; 58 (3): 637–647.

124　*About 50 percent of the variability*: Kalmbach DA, Schneider LD, Cheung J, et al. "Genetic basis of chronotype in humans: insights from three landmark GWAS." *Sleep* 2017; 40 (2): zsw048.

124　*Chronotypes are typically measured*: Levandovski R, Sasso E, Hidalgo MP. "Chronotype: a review of the advances, limits and applicability of the main instruments used in the literature to assess human phenotype." *Trends in Psychiatry and Psychotherapy* 2013; 35: 3–11.

124　*About 60 percent of us have sleep midpoints*: Fischer D, Lombardi DA, Marucci-Wellman H, Roenneberg T. "Chronotypes in the US—influence of age and sex." *PLoS One* 2017; 12 (6): e0178782.

125　*Chronobiologist Dr. Till Roenneberg*: Roenneberg T, Pilz LK, Zerbini G, Winnebeck EC. "Chronotype and social jetlag: a (self-)critical review." *Biology* 2019; 8 (3): 54.

125　*Monday through Friday, teenagers*: Adolescent Sleep Working Group, Committee on Adolescence, and Council on School Health. "School start times for adolescents." *Pediatrics* 2014; 134 (3): 642–649.

125　*and given our cultural favoritism*: Bonke J. "Do morning-type people earn more than evening-type people? how chronotypes influence income." *Annals of Economics and Statistics* 2012; 105/106: 55–72.

125　*Science shows us that we all have little clocks*: "Sleep drive and your body clock." Sleep Foundation. July 28, 2020. sleep foundation.org/articles/sleep-drive-and-your-body-clock.

126　*There are known sex and individual differences*: Santhi N, Lazar AS, McCabe PJ, Lo JC, Groeger JA, Dijk DJ. "Sex differences in the circadian regulation of sleep and waking cognition in humans." *Proceedings of the National Academy of Sciences USA* 2016; 113 (19): E2730–E2739.

126 *Women's clocks also run*: Duffy JF, et al. "Sex difference in the near-24-hour intrinsic period of the human circadian timing system." *Proceedings of the National Academy of Sciences USA* 2011; 108 (Suppl 3): 15602–15608.

126 *This disorder, which afflicts about*: Nesbitt AD. "Delayed sleep-wake phase disorder." *Journal of Thoracic Disease* 2018; 10 (Suppl 1): S103–S111.

128 *Research has shown that couples who are mismatched*: Larson JH, Crane DR, Smith CW. "Morning and night couples: the effect of wake and sleep patterns on marital adjustment." *Journal of Marital and Family Therapy* 1991; 17: 53–65.

129 *However, research that my colleagues and I*: Hasler BP, Troxel WM. "Couples' nighttime sleep efficiency and concordance: evidence for bidirectional associations with daytime relationship functioning." *Psychosomatic Medicine* 2010; 72 (8): 794–801.

129 *In one study, led by Heather Gunn*: Gunn HE, Buysse DJ, Hasler BP, Begley A, Troxel WM. "Sleep concordance in couples is associated with relationship characteristics." *Sleep* 2015; 38 (6): 933–939.

130 *In a subsequent study, we found that couples*: Gunn HE, Buysse DJ, Matthews KA, Kline CE, Cribbet MR, Troxel WM. "Sleep-wake concordance in couples is inversely associated with cardiovascular disease risk markers." *Sleep* 2017; 40 (1): zsw028.

130 *In another study, we found that on nights*: Hasler BP, Troxel WM. "Couples' nighttime sleep efficiency and concordance: evidence for bidirectional associations with daytime relationship functioning." *Psychosomatic Medicine* 2010; 72 (8): 794–801.

130 *Research also shows that couples who are mismatched*: Larson JH, Crane DR, Smith CW. "Morning and night couples: the

effect of wake and sleep patterns on marital adjustment." *Journal of Marital and Family Therapy* 1991; 17: 53–65.

130 *Peter joins the roughly fifteen million*: "Job flexibilities and work schedules summary." Economic news release. US Bureau of Labor Statistics. September 24, 2019. bls.gov/news .release/flex2.nr0.htm.

131 *Physicians and other medical workers*: Collier R. "Doctors top list of worst drivers for fifth straight year." *Canadian Medical Association Journal* 2018; 190 (29): E896–E897. Yaghmour NA, Brigham TP, Richter T, et al. "Causes of death of residents in ACGME-accredited programs 2000 through 2014: implications for the learning environment." *Academic Medicine* 2017; 92 (7): 976–983.

132 *Unfortunately, part of our cultural tendency*: Blum AB, Shea S, Czeisler CA, Landrigan CP, Leape L. "Implementing the 2009 Institute of Medicine recommendations on resident physician work hours, supervision, and safety." *Nature and Science of Sleep* 2011; 3: 47–85. Federal Motor Carrier Safety Administration. "Hours of service of drivers: final rule." *Federal Register*. June 1, 2020. federalregister.gov/documents/2020/06/01 /2020-11469/hours-of-service-of-drivers.

136 *Composite Morningness Questionnaire*: Smith CS, Reilly C, Midkiff K. "Evaluation of three circadian rhythm questionnaires with suggestions for an improved measure of morningness." *Journal of Applied Psychology* 1989; 74 (5): 728–738.

CHAPTER 8: IN SICKNESS AND IN HEALTH

143 *evidencing both visible and "invisible" wounds*: Tanielian T, Jaycox KH, eds. *Invisible Wounds of War: Psychological and Cognitive Injuries, Their Consequences, and Services to Assist Recovery*. Santa Monica, CA: RAND, 2008.

143 *As research was conducted*: Plumb TR, Peachey JT, Zelman DC. "Sleep disturbance is common among servicemembers and veterans of Operations Enduring Freedom and Iraqi Freedom." *Psychological Services* 2014; 11 (2): 209–219.

143 *My colleagues and I spent five years*: Brooks Holliday S, Haas A, Shih RA, Troxel WM. "Prevalence and consequences of sleep problems in military wives." *Sleep Health* 2016; 2 (2): 116–122. Fillo J, Brooks Holliday S, DeSantis A, et al. "Observed relationship behaviors and sleep in military veterans and their partners." *Annals of Behavioral Medicine* 2017; 51 (6): 879–889.

145 *As the population in the US*: Stuckler D. "Population causes and consequences of leading chronic diseases: a comparative analysis of prevailing explanations." *Milbank Quarterly* 2008; 86 (2): 273–326.

145 *In fact, national data suggests that sixty-six million*: National Research Council Committee on the Role of Human Factors in Home Health Care. "7: Informal caregivers in the United States: prevalence, caregiver characteristics, and ability to provide care." *The Role of Human Factors in Home Health Care: Workshop Summary*. Washington, DC: National Academies Press, 2010. ncbi.nlm.nih.gov/books/NBK210048/.

145 *Substantial research shows that the health*: Kershaw T, Ellis KR, Yoon H, Schafenacker A, Katapodi M, Northouse L. "The interdependence of advanced cancer patients' and their family caregivers' mental health, physical health, and self-efficacy over time." *Annals of Behavioral Medicine* 2015; 49: 901–911.

145 *With a growing number of Americans*: Kasper JD, Freedman VA, Spillman BC, Wolff JL. "The disproportionate impact of dementia on family and unpaid caregiving to older adults." *Health Affairs* 2015; 34 (10): 1642–1649.

146 *Nighttime caregiving responsibilities*: Gaugler JE, Yu F, Krichbaum K, Wyman JF. "Predictors of nursing home admission for persons with dementia." *Medical Care* 2009; 47 (2): 191–

198. Published correction appears in *Medical Care* 2009; 47 (5): 606.

146 *phenomenon known as "sundowning."*: Khachiyants N, Trinkle D, Son SJ, Kim KY. "Sundown syndrome in persons with dementia: an update." *Psychiatry Investigations* 2011; 8 (4): 275–287.

146 *For example, among the longer-term consequences*: Leggett AN, Morley M, Smagula SF. "'It's been a hard day's night': sleep problems in caregivers for older adults." *Current Sleep Medicine Reports* 2020; 6: 1–10.

146 *A summary of the available literature*: Byun E, Lerdal A, Gay CL, Lee KA. "How adult caregiving impacts sleep: a systematic review." *Current Sleep Medicine Reports* 2016; 2 (4): 191–205.

146 *Caregivers often report*: McCurry SM, Gibbons LE, Logsdon RG, Vitiello MV, Teri L. "Insomnia in caregivers of persons with dementia: who is at risk and what can be done about it?" *Sleep Medicine Clinics* 2009; 4 (4): 519–526.

147 *A commonly used framework*: Spielman AJ, et al. "A behavioral perspective on insomnia treatment." *Psychiatric Clinics of North America* 1987; 10: 541–553.

147 *it's important to identify some underlying vulnerability factors*: Ohayon MM. "Epidemiology of insomnia: what we know and what we still need to learn." *Sleep Medicine Reviews* 2002; 6 (2): 97–111.

147 *Increasing age is also associated*: Li J, Vitiello MV, Gooneratne NS. "Sleep in normal aging." *Sleep Medicine Clinics* 2018; 13 (1): 1–11.

147 *Other predisposing factors*: LeBlanc M, Mérette C, Savard J, Ivers H, Baillargeon L, Morin CM. "Incidence and risk factors of insomnia in a population-based sample." *Sleep* 2009; 32 (8): 1027–1037.

148 *Studies have shown that higher stress levels*: Guastella A, Moulds M. "The impact of rumination on sleep quality

following a stressful life event." *Personality and Individual Differences* 2007; 42: 1151–1162. Hall MH, Casement MD, Troxel WM, et al. "Chronic stress is prospectively associated with sleep in midlife women: the SWAN sleep study." *Sleep* 2015; 38 (10): 1645–1654.

148 *For some, the stress of caregiving*: Schulz R, Sherwood PR. "Physical and mental health effects of family caregiving." *American Journal of Nursing* 2008; 108 (9 Suppl): 23–27.

148 *Sleep problems can also directly lead to depression*: Fernandez-Mendoza J, Shea S, Vgontzas AN, Calhoun SL, Liao D, Bixler EO. "Insomnia and incident depression: role of objective sleep duration and natural history." *Journal of Sleep Research* 2015; 24 (4): 390–398.

150 *These perpetuating factors*: McCurry SM, Logsdon RG, Teri L, Vitiello MV. "Sleep disturbances in caregivers of persons with dementia: contributing factors and treatment implications." *Sleep Medicine Reviews* 2007; 11 (2): 143–153.

151 *One of the most striking demonstrations*: Monk TH, Begley AE, Billy BD, et al. "Sleep and circadian rhythms in spousally bereaved seniors." *Chronobiology International* 2008; 25 (1): 83–98.

151 *Scientists studying circadian rhythms have given a name*: Ehlers CL, Kupfer DJ, Frank E, Monk TH. "Biological rhythms and depression: the role of zeitgebers and zeitstoreres." *Depression* 1993; 1: 285–293.

151 *Research further shows that such inconsistency*: Laird KT, Krause B, Funes C, et al. "Psychobiological factors of resilience and depression in late life." *Translational Psychiatry* 2019; 9 (88). Smagula SF, Hall MH, Stahl ST. "Rest-activity rhythms and depression symptoms in older bereaved adults." *International Psychogeriatrics* 2019; 31 (11): 1675–1676.

151 *Dr. Sarah Stahl is a researcher*: Stahl ST, Emanuel J, Albert SM, et al. "Design and rationale for a technology-based

healthy lifestyle intervention in older adults grieving the loss of a spouse." *Contemporary Clinical Trials Communications* 2017; 8: 99–105. Stahl ST, Schulz R. "Changes in routine health behaviors following late-life bereavement: a systematic review." *Journal of Behavioral Medicine* 2014; 37 (4): 736–755.

152 *One fascinating aspect*: Sarah Stahl, personal communication, January 15, 2020.

154 *"there are only four kinds of people:* "Written testimony of former First Lady Rosalynn Carter before the Senate Special Committee on Aging." Rosalynn Carter Institute for Caregiving. Georgia Southwestern State University. Americus, GA. May 26, 2011. cartercenter.org/news/editorials_speeches /rosalynn-carter-committee-on-aging-testimony.html.

154 *It's called energy generation*: Harvey AG, Eidelman P. "Chapter 8: intervention to reduce unhelpful beliefs about sleep." In Perlis M, Aloia M, Kuhn B, eds., *Behavioral Treatments for Sleep Disorders*. San Diego: Academic Press, 2011. 79–89.

155 *She has pioneered many of the cognitive techniques*: Harvey AG, Sharpley AL, Ree MJ, Stinson K, Clark DM. "An open trial of cognitive therapy for chronic insomnia." *Behaviour Research and Therapy* 2007; 45 (10): 2491–2501.

CHAPTER 9: SNORING AND OTHER SHARED SLEEP STRUGGLES

165 *Across the spectrum of chronic health conditions*: Martire LM, Schulz R, Helgeson VS, Small BJ, Saghafi EM. "Review and meta-analysis of couple-oriented interventions for chronic illness." *Annals of Behavioral Medicine* 2010; 40 (3): 325–342.

166 *Estimates suggest that roughly 10 percent*: Mai E, Buysse DJ. "Insomnia: prevalence, impact, pathogenesis, differential diagnosis, and evaluation." *Sleep Medicine Clinics* 2008; 3 (2): 167–174.

166 *Many of us, however, upward of 30 to 40 percent*: Ohayon MM. "Epidemiology of insomnia: what we know and what we still need to learn." *Sleep Medicine Reviews* 2002; 6 (2): 97–111.

166 *sleep studies, otherwise known as overnight polysomnography*: Sateia MJ. "International classification of sleep disorders— third edition." *Chest* 2014; 146: 1387–1394.

167 *This has been referred to as paradoxical*: Weinberger Y, Kaganovskiy L, Weinstein M. "Sleep state perception: effects of age, gender, and co-existing sleep disorders." *Chest* 2016; 150 (4, Supplement): 1266A.

168 *The good news, in either case, is that CBT-I*: van Straten A, van der Zweerde T, Kleiboer A, Cuijpers P, Morin CM, Lancee J. "Cognitive and behavioral therapies in the treatment of insomnia: a meta-analysis." *Sleep Medicine Reviews* 2018; 38: 3–16.

170 *Given that insomnia is at least, in part, a thought disorder*: Carney CE, Edinger JD, Morin CM, et al. "Examining maladaptive beliefs about sleep across insomnia patient groups." *Journal of Psychosomatic Research* 2010; 68 (1): 57–65.

170 *The problem is that this constant focus on insomnia*: Rogojanski J, Carney CE, Monson CM. "Interpersonal factors in insomnia: a model for integrating bed partners into cognitive behavioral therapy for insomnia." *Sleep Medicine Reviews* 2013; 17 (1): 55–64.

172 *When people start sleeping poorly*: Williams J, Roth A, Vatthauer K, McCrae CS. "Cognitive behavioral treatment of insomnia." *Chest* 2013; 143 (2): 554–565.

172 *Some of the most well-intentioned*: Ellis JG, Deary V, Troxel WM. "The role of perceived partner alliance on the efficacy of CBT-I: preliminary findings from the Partner Alliance in Insomnia Research Study (PAIRS)." *Behavioral Sleep Medicine* 2015; 13 (1): 64–72. Mellor A, Hamill K, Jenkins MM, Baucom DH, Norton PJ, Drummond SPA. "Partner-assisted

cognitive behavioural therapy for insomnia versus cognitive behavioural therapy for insomnia: a randomised controlled trial." *Trials* 2019; 20 (1): 262.

173 *an important but often overlooked criterion of insomnia*: Thorpy MJ. "Classification of sleep disorders." *Neurotherapeutics* 2012; 9 (4): 687–701.

173 *This is an important distinction*: Komada Y, Inoue Y, Hayashida K, Nakajima T, Honda M, Takahashi K. "Clinical significance and correlates of behaviorally induced insufficient sleep syndrome." *Sleep Medicine* 2008; 9 (3): 851–856.

173 *Therefore, one of the most powerful behavioral*: Morin CM, Bootzin RR, Buysse DJ, Edinger JD, Espie CA, Lichstein KL. "Psychological and behavioral treatment of insomnia: update of the recent evidence (1998–2004)." *Sleep* 2006; 29: 1398–1414.

174 *As simple as this strategy sounds*: Kyle SD, Miller CB, Rogers Z, Siriwardena AN, Macmahon KM, Espie CA. "Sleep restriction therapy for insomnia is associated with reduced objective total sleep time, increased daytime somnolence, and objectively impaired vigilance: implications for the clinical management of insomnia disorder." *Sleep* 2014; 37 (2): 229–237.

174 *If you ever took an introductory*: Colomb J, Brembs B. "The biology of psychology." *Communicative & Integrative Biology* 2010; 3 (2): 142–145.

175 *From a treatment perspective, stimulus control*: Bootzin R, Epstein D. "Understanding and treating insomnia." *Annual Review of Clinical Psychology* 2006; 7: 435–458.

176 *The technique of stimulus control*: Troxel WM, Germain A, Buysse DJ. "Clinical management of insomnia with brief behavioral treatment (BBTI)." *Behavioral Sleep Medicine* 2012; 10 (4): 266–279.

178 *This scenario plays out in roughly*: Peppard PE, Young T, Barnet JH, et al. "Increased prevalence of sleep-disordered

breathing in adults." *American Journal of Epidemiology* 2013; 177 (9): 1006–1014.

179   *OSA and its primary symptom of loud snoring*: Osman AM, Carter SG, Carberry JC, Eckert DJ. "Obstructive sleep apnea: current perspectives." *Nature and Science of Sleep* 2018; 10: 21–34.

179   *OSA has been called a "disease of listeners"*: Schmaling KB, Afari N. "Couples coping with respiratory illness." In Schmaling KB, Scher TG, eds. *The Psychology of Couples and Illness: Theory, Research, and Practice*. Washington, DC: American Psychological Association, 2000. 71–104.

179   *They experience the profound consequences*: Luyster FS. "Impact of obstructive sleep apnea and its treatments on partners: a literature review." *Journal of Clinical Sleep Medicine* 2017; 13 (3): 467–477.

179   *Women sleeping with snorers are three*: Ulfberg J, Carter N, Talback M, Edling C. "Adverse health effects among women living with heavy snorers." *Health Care for Women International* 2000; 21 (2): 81–90.

179   *Studies further suggest that if you sleep with a snorer*: Beninati W, Harris CD, Herold DL, Shepard JW Jr. "The effect of snoring and obstructive sleep apnea on the sleep quality of bed partners." *Mayo Clinic Proceedings*. 1999; 74 (10): 955–958. Sardesai MG, Tan AK, Fitzpatrick M. "Noise-induced hearing loss in snorers and their bed partners." *Journal of Otolaryngology* 2003; 32 (3): 141–145.

180   *Estimates suggest that anywhere between*: National Sleep Foundation. *2005 Sleep in America Poll*. Washington, DC: National Sleep Foundation, 2005.

181   *Despite the fact that snoring*: Blumen M, Quera Salva MA, d'Ortho M-P, et al. "Effect of sleeping alone on sleep quality in female bed partners of snorers." 2009; 34 (5): 1127–1131.

181   *Several years ago, I had the opportunity*: Troxel W. "Sleep and couples: for better or worse, day AND night?" ABC News. May 20, 2013. abcnews.go.com/blogs/health/2013/05/20/sleep-and-couples-for-better-or-worse-day-and-night.

182   *There is good news*: Calik MW. "Treatments for obstructive sleep apnea." *Journal of Clinical Outcomes Management* 2016; 23 (4): 181–192. Luyster FS. "Impact of obstructive sleep apnea and its treatments on partners: a literature review." *Journal of Clinical Sleep Medicine* 2017; 13 (3): 467–477. Zheng D, Xu Y, You S, et al. "Effects of continuous positive airway pressure on depression and anxiety symptoms in patients with obstructive sleep apnoea: results from the Sleep Apnoea Cardiovascular Endpoint randomised trial and meta-analysis." *EClinicalMedicine* 2019; 11: 89–96.

182   *Studies have shown that, after successful treatment*: Luyster FS. "Impact of obstructive sleep apnea." Parish JM, Lyng PJ. "Quality of life in bed partners of patients with obstructive sleep apnea or hypopnea after treatment with continuous positive airway pressure." *Chest* 2003; 124 (3): 942–947.

182   *Fifty percent of individuals prescribed*: Lin H, Prasad AS, Pan CG, Rowley JA. "Factors associated with noncompliance to treatment with positive airway pressure." *Archives of Otolaryngology—Head & Neck Surgery* 2007; 133 (1): 69–72.

182   *Other treatments exist*: Calik MW. "Treatments for obstructive sleep apnea."

183   *My colleague Dr. Kelly Baron*: Baron KG, Gunn HE, Wolfe LF, et al. "Relationships and CPAP adherence among women with obstructive sleep apnea." *Sleep Science Practice* 2017; 1 (10). Baron KG, Gunn HE, Czajkowski LA, Smith TW, Jones CR. "Spousal involvement in CPAP: does pressure help?" *Journal of Clinical Sleep Medicine* 2012; 8 (2): 147–153.

184   *Narcolepsy is thought of as*: Burgess CR, Scammell TE. "Narcolepsy: neural mechanisms of sleepiness and cataplexy." *Journal of Neuroscience* 2012; 32 (36): 12305–12311.

184   *Cataplexy is usually triggered*: Schiappa C, Scarpelli S, D'Atri A, et al. "Narcolepsy and emotional experience: a review of the literature." *Behavioral and Brain Functions* 2018; 14 (19).

185   *Narcolepsy is a relatively uncommon disorder*: "Narcolepsy fact sheet." National Institute of Neurological Disorders and Stroke. NIH Publication No. 17-1637. ninds.nih.gov/disorders /patient-caregiver-education/fact-sheets/narcolepsy-fact-sheet. Accessed September 10, 2020.

186   *Not surprisingly, individuals with narcolepsy*: Bruck D. "The impact of narcolepsy on psychological health and role behaviors: negative effects and comparisons with other illness groups." *Sleep Medicine* 2001; 2: 437–446.

186   *RLS is a neurological disorder*: Ohayon MM, O'Hara R, Vitiello MV. "Epidemiology of restless legs syndrome: A synthesis of the literature." *Sleep Medicine Reviews* 2012; 16: 283–295.

186   *The primary symptom of RLS*: Hornyak M, Scholz H, Kohnen R, Bengel J, Kassubek J, Trenkwalder C. "What treatment works best for restless legs syndrome? meta-analyses of dopaminergic and non-dopaminergic medications." *Sleep Medicine Reviews* 2014; 18 (2): 153–164. Published correction appears in *Sleep Medicine Reviews* 2014; 18 (4): 367–368.

187   *Recent study of RLS*: Ondo W. "Restless legs syndrome: 'Patient Odyssey' survey of disease burden on patient and spouses/partners." *Sleep Medicine* 2018; 47: 51–53.

187   *The major difference between parasomnias*: Markov D, Jaffe F, Doghramji K. "Update on parasomnias: a review for psychiatric practice." *Psychiatry (Edgmont)* 2006; 3 (7): 69–76.

187   *The good and the bad news is that RBD*: Khawaja I, Spurling BC, Singh S. "REM Sleep Behavior Disorder." StatPearls. June 29, 2020. ncbi.nlm.nih.gov/books/NBK534239.

CHAPTER 10: NEGOTIATING THE NIGHT

198 *Research shows that endings are important*: Schwörer B, Krott NR, Oettingen G. "Saying goodbye and saying it well: Consequences of a (not) well-rounded ending." *Motivation Science* 2020; 6 (1): 21–33.

Acknowledgments

IT'S DAY NUMBER HELL-IF-I-KNOW OF STAY-AT-HOME ORDERS during the COVID-19 pandemic, and to put it bluntly, the day started out rather bleak. I woke with the feeling of "here we go again, another day of not seeing friends, of sharing my home office space with my two teenagers and my husband, and of thinking, *How long will this last? And how will we ever recover from this?*" Per usual, I allow myself about ten minutes of wallowing; then I force myself out of bed and start being my own therapist. When things get rough: (1) get out of bed, (2) focus on the present, (3) do something that gives you pleasure or a sense of mastery (accomplishment), and (4) practice gratitude. So here I sit, out of bed (albeit in pajamas), already feeling better because I am actually doing something on my to-do list, and reflecting on the many people and entities who have made this book possible and given me the amazing opportunity to share some knowledge and, if I may be so bold, to make a difference in some people's lives. These are the words on my dearly departed father's gravestone: "He made a difference." To me, they're words to live by, if only aspirational.

As a scientist, I am deeply indebted to the multidisciplinary research community, including sleep scientists, historians, sociologists, relationship researchers, and others, whose work is highlighted in this book and has shaped my program of research over the past fifteen years. I would like to specifically acknowledge my two primary research mentors, Dr. Karen A. Matthews and Dr. Daniel J. Buysse, who supported my independence and encouraged me to pursue my somewhat "out there" idea (at the time) that studying sleep in the context of couples was an avenue worthy of pursuit. I would also like to acknowledge the work of specific researchers who graciously agreed to be interviewed for this book, including Dr. Marco Hafner, Dr. Roger Ekirch, Dr. Amie Gordon, Dr. Sarah Stahl, Dr. Robert Meadows, Dr. Kelly Baron, Dr. Debra Umberson, Dr. Douglas Teti, and Dr. Sarah Burgard. Special thanks to my colleagues, including Sonni Efron, Dr. Regina Shih, Dr. Susan Strauss, Dr. Alice Gregory, and Dr. Rebecca Robbins for providing astute and honest feedback on earlier drafts of this manuscript. As a clinician, I am deeply indebted to my clients over the years, whose stories and experiences (all anonymized in this book) give meaning to the work I do and keep me focused on why I do the work: to make people's lives better by improving their sleep and the quality of their relationships—both pillars of health and well-being.

One of the great things about practicing gratitude is it teaches you to be humble and also realize that you are not alone, even in the most challenging times. There were many occasions while writing

Acknowledgments

this book when I felt overwhelmed and uncertain of where to go next. I am indebted to my writing coach and friend, Tom Godfrey, who has been with me every step of the way, to help me find better ways to translate research findings to a broader audience and to bring life to the stories described herein. I am also thankful to my agent, Ted Weinstein, for taking a chance with me as I embarked on my first book and for Dan Ambrosio and the publishing team at Hachette Go, who have provided support, feedback, and guidance throughout this process.

On the personal front, I am deeply blessed with family and friends who are my lifeblood, my greatest source of strength and motivation, and my greatest source of joy and comfort. To my wonderful friends, thank you for checking in on me and how the book was coming along, providing the encouragement I needed along the way, and offering your stories of shared sleep joys and challenges. To my mother and late father, I would like to thank you both for giving me the best example of the power of a healthy relationship and the meaning of resilience. And to my husband, Jon, and our two children, Jack and Calla, thank you for making this a life worth living. You are my reason for being and my most cherished gifts.

Like any good scientist, I am now doing a pre- and post-evaluation of myself following this exercise in gratitude, and guess what? I feel a heck of a lot better than when I started this exercise this morning. I feel lighter, happier, and ready to attack this day (even if it feels very much like yesterday). I have no doubt that we as a society have many challenging days ahead of us as we work through the aftermath and ongoing challenges associated with the COVID-19 pandemic as well as the many other challenges we face in our deeply divided country, but I hope you will find in these pages some strategies that will give you a better sense of control and of hope and better strategies to cope even during difficult times, as a good night of sleep and having a partner to rely on are two of the most important cornerstones of resilience.

Be well. Sleep well. Love heartily.